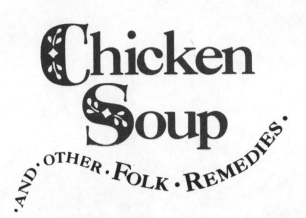

Chicken Soup

· AND · OTHER · FOLK · REMEDIES ·

Chicken Soup

AND · OTHER · FOLK · REMEDIES ·

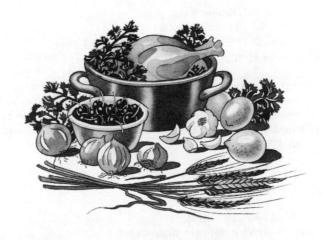

JOAN WILEN AND LYDIA WILEN

Fawcett Columbine · New York

Chicken Soup and Other Folk Remedies
is dedicated to the loving memory of
Lillian and Jack Wilen—
Mom, who made the best chicken soup
in the whole wide world!
and Dad, who insisted we wear
camphor squares around our necks!

A Fawcett Columbine Book
Published by Ballantine Books
Copyright © 1984 by Joan Wilen and Lydia Wilen
Illustrations copyright © 1984 by Elizabeth Koda-Callan

Library of Congress Catalog Card Number: 84-90842
ISBN 0-449-90109-2

Designed by Beth Tondreau
Cover design by Georgia Morrissey
Cover illustration by Elizabeth Koda-Callan

Manufactured in the United States of America
First Edition: November 1984
10 9 8 7 6 5 4 3 2 1

Contents

Acknowledgments

A big Thank You to all the people who offered us their loving support, good wishes, and remedies:

Harry Wilen, Betty and Morris Wilen, Mina and Hy Wilen, Ann and Linda Iris Wilen, Roger Yager, Laura Yager, Dr. Ann Wigmore, Mary Pat Werner, Robert Weinstein, Gene, Anne and Theresa Vilfordi, Chris Verveniotis, Gwen Verdon, Judy Twersky, Vita Thalrose, Thelma Taylor, Margaret Sunshine, David Stanford, Esther Spitzer, Bill Smiddy, Rudy Shur, Gloria and Sidney R. Seltzer, Michael Sedgwick, Ellen and Fred Schreiber, Priscilla Schmidt, Johnny Saltos, Dr. Norman and Susan Ruttner, Hilda and Moses Rosner, Patricia Riley, Rev. Thomas J. Ralph, Chipp Prosnit, Richard Perozzi, Eileen Pinsker, Ann and Joe Paull, Robert Pardi, Diana Okula, Eileen Nock, George Nider, Martha Neag, Dr. Marie Neag, John Nathan, Judy Montague, Blanche Miller, Bill McHugh, Frank McHale, Nick Malekos, Sheila Lukins, Countess Bianca Lovatelli, Gary Louisa, Mia Lottringer, Randie Levine, Paul David Levine, Mimi Levine, Ruth Lesser, Wendy and Jonathon Lazear, Ruth Landa, Helen and Larry Koster, Minnie Koskowitz, Jane and Bill Katz, Arleen and Anthony Kane, Lilly and Lester Kahn, Dr. Ronald N. Jones, Gene Stanley Jones, Eric Stephen Jacobs, Sylvia Holzberg, Dr. Ronald Hoffman, Suki, Elaine, Tina and Hy Hill, Werner Haas, Libby Gurian, Veerani Gunavardhana, Mary Lynn and Howard Gottfried, Frances Goldstein, Barry Goldsmith, Walter Gidaly, Ronald E. Franzmeier, Vic Fiore, Thelma Felcher, Ray and Charles Farin, Rev. Lee Domez, B.J. DeSimone,

Naomi Davis, James Daniels, Dorothy Conway, Becky and Brian Clement, James Chotas, Fung Wing Chin, Diana Chesmel, Morrie Buttnick, Miles P. Burton, Patricia Burke, Helen Burgess, Mildred Borofsky, Hank Blumfarb, Bill Mason Bivens, France Anthony Benko, Marlene Hope Ascherman, Sheila Anderson and Mollie Adler.

Special Thanks to Mary Ellen Pinkham, to whom we will always be grateful for giving us our first chance.

For giving us *this* chance, Extra Special Thanks to the woman we're proud to have as our editor, Leona Nevler. Thanks also to Joelle Delbourgo for caring about this project, and to Michelle Russell and Beth Heinsohn. All of you have helped to make this book-writing business a lovely experience.

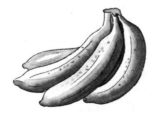

Introduction

As soon as we signed the contract for *Chicken Soup and Other Folk Remedies*, we went to all our relatives, asking for their home remedies. We heard wonderful "old-country" stories about remarkable cures, but times and places have changed dramatically. Going to the outskirts of Lomza Gubernia in Russia-Poland to pick *bopka blettles* is no longer practical. And we knew we wanted this book to not only be SAFE and EFFECTIVE, but PRACTICAL, too.

Yes, PRACTICAL! Every herb, fruit, vegetable, vitamin, mineral and liquid—in fact, all the ingredients mentioned in the book— can be bought at your local health food store, supermarket or green grocer— that is, if they aren't already in your home.

Our directions are easy to follow and, for the most part, specific. If exact amounts are not indicated, it means we could not find them, but we thought the remedy was important enough to include. Please use common sense and listen to your body every step of the way.

That brings us to an important point—this book's being SAFE. It is if you consult a medical authority before starting any self-help health care treatment.

We (Wilen sisters) are not medical authorities. The closest either of us comes is that Joan used to date a pharmacist and Lydia's favorite playwright is Doc Simon.

Please, for your own well-being, heed the NOTES throughout the book. They stress the fact that our home-remedy suggestions are scientifically unproven and should not take the place of professional health care that may be needed for certain ailments and for persistent symptoms. Effective proven medical treatment is available for almost all conditions mentioned in this book. You can use the remedies in addition to, but not as a substitute for, professional help.

How EFFECTIVE are the remedies? It's as though our parents saw the future when they named us. Lydia is named after our mother's aunt, who was the town herbalist/midwife. Joan is named for our father's cousin, the town hypochondriac. It worked out swell. As we researched and wrote each chapter, Joan would get symptoms, and we got the chance to try lots of remedies. The ones with which we don't have first-hand experience come highly recommended, usually by more than one source. We've reasoned it out: The remedies that work have been passed down from generation to generation, and the ones that didn't work most likely haven't survived the trip here.

While not all the remedies will be cure-alls for everyone, they're worth a try, and as grandma used to say, "It wouldn't hurt!" (Actually, our grandmother used to say, "It vouldn't hoit!")

Since you seem to be interested in home remedies, we would love your input. Have you tried any of these remedies? What has been your experience with them?

Do you have any of your own remedies you would

like to share with us? We can be reached by mail, in care of the publisher.

Thank you for reading our book.

To your health!*

Joan Wilen and Lydia Wilen
c/o FAWCETT BOOKS
201 East 50th Street
New York, N.Y. 10022

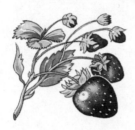

*Gëzuar! (Albanian) Fi schettak! (Arabian) Genatzt! (Armenian) Prosit! (Austria) Op uw gezonheid! (Belgian) Naz dar! (Bohemian) Viva! (Brazilian) Yum sen! (Chinese) Na Zdravi! (Czechoslavakian) Skål! (Norwegian, Swedish, and Danish) Proost! (Dutch) Je zia sano! (Esperanto) Kippis! (Finnish) A votre santé! (French) Auf ihr wohol! (German) Eis Igian! (Greek) Kasûgta! (Greenlandic) Okole maluna! (Hawaiian) Kedves egeszsegere! (Hungarian) Santanka nu! (Icelandic) Jaikind! (Indian) Selámat! (Indonesian) Besalmati! (Iranian) A la salute! (Italian) Kampai! (Japanese) Kong gang ul wi ha yo! (Korean) I sveikas! (Lithuanian) Slamat minum! (Malayan) Salud! (Spanish) Saha wa'afiab! (Moroccan) Kia ora! (New Zealand) Zanda bashi (Pakistani) Mabuhay! (Philippine) Noroc! (Rumanian) Na zdorovia! (Russian) Sawasdi! (Thai) Şerefe! (Turkish) Boovatje zdorovi! (Ukrainian) Iechyd da! (Welsh) Tsu gezunt! (Yiddish) Zivio! (Yugoslavian) Oogy wawa! (Zulu)

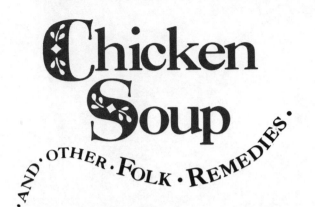

Chicken Soup
AND · OTHER · FOLK · REMEDIES ·

The Home-Remedy StarterKit

‡ ALFALFA

This easy-to-sprout seed (see "Preparation Guide" for sprouting instructions) is very high in protein and has phosphorus, iron, potassium, vitamins A, E, K, B-8, D and U. It is also rich in calcium. What more can we say? "Pass the alfalfa, please."

‡ APPLE CIDER VINEGAR

A bottle of apple cider vinegar is a must for your Home-Remedy Starter Kit. It has been said to help a wide variety of conditions from top to bottom—sore throats to diaper rash.

‡ BARLEY

Hippocrates, the Father of Medicine, felt that everyone should drink barley water daily to maintain good health. Barley is rich in iron and vitamin B. It is said to help prevent tooth decay and hair loss, improve fingernails and toenails, and help heal ulcers, diarrhea, and bronchial spasms. (See "Preparation Guide" for barley water recipe.)

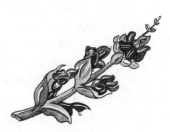

‡ CAMOMILE

This herb, rich in calcium and potassium, is said to be wonderful for helping heal nervous disorders, sleeplessness, menstrual problems and stomachaches. You can buy camomile loose or in tea-bag form.

‡ CAYENNE PEPPER

This herb is said to be nature's stimulant, stopper, cleanser, heater and healer. It's important for all kinds of first aid. As a condiment, it helps bring out flavor in food. Cayenne pepper is strong and takes some getting used to. NEVER exceed recommended dosage.

‡ GARLIC

Garlic has been used to help heal just about every ailment except bad breath. There is a fan club for garlic groupies. It's called "Lovers of the Stinking Rose." Eat garlic raw, use it as a spice in cooking and take garlic pills or capsules. If the pills and capsules repeat on you and you find it unpleasant, you can get deodorized garlic capsules. Fortunately, the substance that gives garlic its potent smell does not have very much to do with the bulb's healing properties.

CAUTION: While garlic may be helpful and healing to many, there are some people whose stomachs are tortured by it. Most likely, you know if you are one of those people. Anyone with an unfavorable reaction to garlic (or any ingredient mentioned in this book), should steer clear of it. We offer a variety of alternative treatments for each ailment.

‡ HONEY

The sugar in honey is in a predigested form, allowing the body to assimilate it quickly. Honey is said to increase calcium retention and rejuvenate the female reproductive system. Some folk medicine followers have used honey in the treatment of asthma, hay fever, allergies, digestive problems, arthritis, hemorrhoids, cuts and wounds, bad complexions, and coughs and colds.

Raw, unprocessed honey has been extracted by centrifugal force and has not been heated or cooked. Heating or cooking may destroy some of the honey's reputed health-giving properties. If you cannot get raw, unprocessed honey, commercially processed honey is better than no honey at all.

CAUTION: NEVER GIVE HONEY TO A CHILD LESS THAN ONE YEAR OLD! Spores found in honey have been linked to botulism in babies.

‡ HORSERADISH

This valuable concentrated food is said to be excellent for sinusitis, stimulating the appetite and aiding in digestion. Prepare your own by grating a fresh horseradish root with an equal amount of lemon juice. Or you can buy prepared horseradish at the grocery store.

‡ LEMON

After researching the use of lemons, a German and English team of physicians concluded that using lemons every day may prolong one's life. Lemons have the highest vitamin C content of all citrus fruits. They are also rich in calcium, potassium and magnesium. Though lemons are acidic, it is said that their effect on the blood is alkalizing. While studying folklore, we saw that lemons were used extensively in treating a wide array of ailments, so much so that they were once considered more of a medicine than a food.

Choose lemons that are thin-skinned and heavy. They are the juiciest.

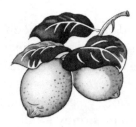

‡ ONION

The onion is in the same plant family as garlic and is almost as versatile. The ancient Egyptians looked at the onion as the symbol of the universe. It has been regarded as a universal healing food, used to treat earaches, colds, fever, wounds, diarrhea, insomnia, warts, and the list goes on. It is believed that a cut onion in a sickroom disinfects the air as it absorbs the germs in that room. Half an onion will help absorb the smell of a just-painted room. With that in mind, never use a cut piece of onion that has been in the kitchen for more than a day.

‡ PARSLEY

Parsley is especially nutritious—high in iron, vitamins A and C, manganese and copper. Don't just decorate a dish with it! For full food value, eat raw parsley, and if you have a juicer, drink parsley juice. It is said to be good for the blood, the bladder and the breath.

‡ POTATO

Raw, peeled, boiled, grated and mashed potatoes; potato water; and potato poultices all help heal, according to American, English and Irish folk medicine. In fact, a popular nineteenth-century Irish saying was "Only two things in this world are too serious to be jested on—potatoes and matrimony." Potatoes are high in protein, vitamins A and B and alkaline salts that are said to help neutralize acid wastes in the body. To get the most nutritional value from eating a potato, boil it whole with the skin on. You lose about one-third of the potato's nutrients when you cut it before you cook it. It is not advisable to eat potatoes that have begun to sprout or potatoes that have been in sunlight and have turned green.

‡ SAUERKRAUT

Sauerkraut is fermented cabbage that has been a popular folk medicine throughout the world for centuries. The lactic acid in sauerkraut is said to encourage the growth of friendly bacteria and help destroy enemy bacteria in the large intestine (where many people believe disease may begin) and in other parts of the digestive tract. Sauerkraut is rich in vitamin B-6—which is important for brain and nervous system functions—and high in calcium—for healthy teeth and bones. In fact, in the hills of West Germany, it is reported that sauerkraut is used as a snack for children, to help prevent tooth decay and heal bad skin conditions. You can make your own sauerkraut (see "Preparation Guide"), or you can buy it in health food or ethnic stores, out of a barrel. The sauerkraut that comes in cans has been processed, and the valuable properties may have been destroyed in the process. For the same reason you should eat sauerkraut at room temperature or cook it over a very low flame. Overheating may destroy the lactic acid and enzymes.

‡ YOGURT

Everyone should be aware of the benefits of eating yogurt, particularly those who take antibiotics. Since antibiotics may kill off healthful bacteria as well as disease-bearing ones, the *Lactobacillus acidophilus* bacteria in yogurt helps counteract the side effects of antibiotics by replacing the friendly bacteria that the chemical remedy may have destroyed. Antibiotics may also cause your skin to be dry, scaly and itchy. Yogurt to the rescue, replacing the intestinal bacteria that produce the B vitamin, biotin, to help clear up the skin condition. Yogurt is rich in B-12, which is good for the nervous system. Yogurt is also said to be an excellent skin cleanser, neutralizer of acidic conditions, an aid in digestion and assimilation of the food we eat, a dysentery preventer and an effective douche.

You can buy yogurt or make it yourself. The advantage of homemade yogurt is that you have control and can produce yogurt with a stronger bacteria culture than the store-bought variety. Health food stores have yogurt starter kits and machines with instructions. If you buy yogurt, stick with the plain kind. Read the ingredients and steer clear of the brands with lots of sugar and artificial flavoring and color. Make sure the yogurt you buy contains active or live cultures.

‡ ACE BANDAGE, GAUZE, CHEESECLOTH, COTTON PADS, STERILE BANDAGES

All of the above are for holding things in place, dabbing things on, making poultices and protecting the skin (for instance, if you have super-sensitive skin, you may want to place gauze between a crushed clove of garlic and your delicate skin). When covering an open cut or wound, use a sterile bandage. If none is available, use a white cotton strip of cloth rather than dyed synthetics.

Preparation Guide

‡ POULTICES

Poultices are usually made with vegetables, fruit or herbs that are minced, chopped, grated, crushed, mashed and sometimes cooked. These ingredients are then wrapped in a clean fabric—cheesecloth, white cotton, muslin—and then applied externally to the affected area.

A poultice is said to be effective when moist. After a few hours, when the poultice dries out, it should be changed—the cloth as well as the ingredients.

Whenever possible, use fresh fruits, vegetables or herbs. If these are unavailable, then use dried herbs. To soften the herb, pour hot water over it. Do not let it steep in boiling water. The herb can lose its effectiveness, particularly in the case of comfrey.

Comfrey poultices seem to be the ones most often used. Comfrey is also called knitbone because from the time of the Crusaders, the leaves were used for repairing and drawing fractured bone segments back together. To make a comfrey poultice, cut a piece of cloth twice the size of the area it will cover. If you're using a fresh leaf, wash it with cool water, then crush it in your hand. Place the leaf on one-half of the cloth and fold over the other half. If you are making a poultice with dried comfrey root and leaves (available in most healthfood stores), pour hot water over the herb, then place the softened herb on half of the cloth, fold over the other half and apply it to the affected body part. Put an Ace bandage or another strip of cloth around the poultice to hold it in place.

‡ BARLEY WATER

Boil 2 ounces of barley in 6 cups of water until there's about half the water—3 cups—left in the pot. Strain. If necessary, add honey and lemon to taste.

‡ MILKING A COCONUT

You need an ice pick or a screwdriver (Phillips, if possible), and a hammer. The coconut has three little black eye-like bald spots on it. Place the ice pick or screwdriver in the middle of one black spot, then hammer the end of it so that it pierces the coconut. Repeat the procedure with the other two black spots and then pour out the coconut milk. The hammer alone should then do the trick on the rest of the coconut. Watch your fingers!

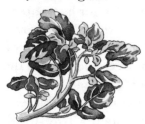

‡ GENERAL RECIPE FOR HERB TEAS

Place a teaspoonful of the herb, or a tea bag, in a glass or ceramic cup and pour boiling water over it. (The average water-to-herb ratio is 1 cup of water to 1 teaspoonful of herb.) Let the herb steep for 5 to 10 minutes, until it's cool enough to drink. Then, strain, sweeten with raw, unprocessed honey (never with sugar, because it negates the value of most herbs) and drink slowly.

‡ DRY ROASTING SUNFLOWER SEEDS

Place a handful of shelled, unprocessed sunflower seeds in a pan, over a low flame. Stay with them for the 2-or-so minutes it takes for them to roast. Jiggle them along the way so that both sides get done. When you hear them crackle and see several of them move by themselves, they're ready. Dry roasting takes out some of the oil and makes the seeds remarkably flavorful. Wait for them to cool off before eating. (We tried this dry-roasting method with pumpkin seeds. They get a little wild, exploding and jumping all over. It's fun but not too practical.)

‡ SPROUTING ALFALFA SEEDS

You're going to need alfalfa seeds, a 1-quart jar, a rubber band for the neck of the jar, nylon mesh or cheesecloth and a dish rack or some kind of stand.

Fill the jar halfway with lukewarm water, preferably filtered. Soak 3 tablespoonsful of alfalfa seeds in the jar overnight (anywhere from 5 to 8 hours).

Put the mesh or cheesecloth over the mouth of the jar, securing it with the rubber band. After the soaking, pour out the water. Turn the jar upside down and at a 45° angle, resting it on the dish rack or stand, making sure the jar's opening allows air in and is not completely covered up by seeds. Let it stand in a dark area. Twice a day (about every 12 hours), fill the jar with cool water, giving the seeds a good rinse, then pour out the water and continue letting it drain in the dark until the next rinse cycle.

When the sprouts are about 1¼ inches long (after 3, 4 or 5 days), put them in the sun or under a grow-light for a day and watch them turn green as they manufacture chlorophyll.

To harvest the sprouts, place them in a bowl, basin or sink filled with water. The hulls will rise to the surface. Scoop off the hulls and put the hull-less sprouts back in the jar, turned upside down to allow the excess water to drain off. Once that happens, they're ready to be eaten and/or refrigerated. They will keep fresh several days.

Alfalfa sprouts are rich in vitamins A, B, C, D, E, F and K; minerals; and amino acids. One pound of seed makes approximately 8 pounds of sprouts.

Sprouting is a lot less complicated than the instructions sound. Once you get into it, you might want to try sprouting mung beans, lentils, radish, fenugreek and chick peas.

According to some medical experts and nutritional researchers, sprouts come as close to being the "perfect food" as anything available.

‡ SAUERKRAUT

1 large head of white cabbage (about 8 cups when shredded)

8 teaspoonsful of sea salt

1 tablespoonful of caraway seeds or fresh or dried dill (OPTIONAL)

1 large container (earthenware crock, glass bowl or stainless steel cookware)

A cover or plate that fits snugly inside the above container

A brick or stones or any 10-pound weight that's clean

A cloth or towel that will fit over the container

Remove the large loose outer leaves of the cabbage, rinse them and leave them for later. Core and finely shred the rest of the cabbage. Spread a layer of cabbage (about 1 cup) on the bottom of the container. Sprinkle the layer with a teaspoonful of sea salt and a few caraway seeds or dill. Repeat layering with cabbage, salt and seeds, ending with a layer of salt. Place those loose outer leaves of cabbage over the top layer. Then, press the cabbage down with the plate or cover and place the weight on top of it. Cover the entire container with a cloth or towel and set it aside in a warm place for 7 to 12 days, depending on how strong you like your sauerkraut.

After a week or more, remove the weight and the plate. Throw away the leaves on top and skim off the yukky-looking mold from the top layer. Transfer the sauerkraut from the container to glass jars with lids, and refrigerate. It should keep for about a month.

Remedies

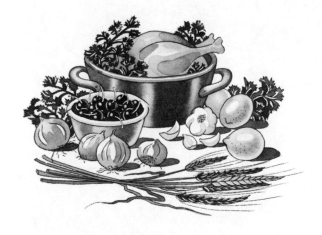

‡Alcoholism

Drinking in excess can make you look wrinkled and haggard, can destroy vital organs and, in general, ruin your life. We know someone who read so much about the bad effects of drinking that he gave up reading.

But seriously... For the problem drinker, we strongly recommend the leading self-help organization for combating alcoholism: Alcoholics Anonymous. Check the white pages of the telephone book for your local chapter.

This section deals with the social drinker who, occasionally, has one too many.

‡ SOBERING UP

The following remedies can help sober up people —that is, make them more alert and communicative. However, *do not trust or depend on those people's reflexes*, especially behind the wheel of a car.

To start with, if a drunk person imagines that the room is spinning, have him or her lie down on a bed and put one foot on the floor to stop that feeling.

To help sober up an intoxicated person, try feeding him or her cucumber—as much as he or she is willing to eat. The cuke's enzyme, erepsin, may dramatically lessen the effect of alcohol.

Honey contains fructose, which promotes the chemical breakdown of alcohol. Give a drunk person a teaspoonful of honey every few minutes. Within 24 hours, and 2 pounds of honey, a person may go from absolutely blotto to being able to 'walk the chalk.'

Try sobering up someone who's tipsy by massaging the tip of his or her nose.

CAUTION: Stimulation of the tip of the nose can cause vomiting, so don't stand right in front of the person you're sobering up.

‡ HANGOVERS

Hangovers can be caused by an allergy or sensitivity to something you drank. Put 1 drop of that drink in a glass of water. Take 3 sips of it. If the hangover symptoms do not disappear within 5 minutes, then drink the rest of the glass of water. If you still don't feel better within a few minutes, then your hangover is not allergy-caused. Try some other remedy.

For the morning after the night before, take ⅛ teaspoonful of cayenne pepper in a glass of water.

According to the Chinese, a cup of ginger tea will help settle an unsettled stomach caused by a hangover. To relieve eye, ear, mouth, nose and brain pain from the hangover, they recommend kneading the fleshy part of the hand between the thumb and the

index finger on both hands. For the pounding hangover headache, massage each thumb, just below the
knuckles.

Take 1 tablespoonful of honey every minute for 5
minutes. Repeat the procedure ½ hour later.

Rub ¼ lemon on each armpit. That may ease the
discomfort of a hangover.

If you really need to recover rapidly from a hangover, go to your local doctor, dentist or hospital and,
under medical supervision, take 10 snorts of oxygen.

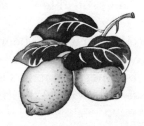

‡Arthritis (Rheumatism, Bursitis, Gout), Muscle Aches, Pains and Sprains

One authority in the field feels that arthritis is a catchall term that includes rheumatism, bursitis and gout. Another specialist believes that arthritis is a form of rheumatism. Still another claims there is no such ailment as rheumatism, that it's a term for several diseases, including arthritis.

No matter what it's called, everyone agrees on two things: Oh, the pain! and all these conditions (herein bunched under the heading of "Arthritis"), involve inflammation of connective tissue of one or more joints.

Knowledge is power! Check your local library for books on arthritis (and there are lots of them). Learn about non-chemical treatments and low-acid diets. There are foods that have been classified as nightshade foods. White potatoes, eggplants, green peppers, and tomatoes are the most common ones and may contribute to the pain of some arthritis sufferers. Consider being professionally tested for a sensitivity to the nightshade foods. Work with a health professional to evaluate your condition and to help you find safe, sensible methods of treatment for relief.

Here are remedies that have been said to be successful for many arthritis sufferers—that is, former arthritis sufferers. These remedies are not substitutions for professional medical treatment.

‡ ARTHRITIS

Cherries are said to be effective because they seem to help prevent crystallization of uric acid and to reduce the uric acid levels in the blood. It is also said that cherries have been known to help the arthritic bumps on knuckles disappear.

EAT CHERRIES! any kind—sweet or sour, fresh, canned or frozen, black, Royal Anne or Bing. DRINK CHERRY JUICE! available without preservatives or sugar added, and also in a concentrated form at health food stores.

One source says to eat cherries and drink the juice throughout the day for 4 days, then stop for 4 days and then start all over again. Another source says to eat up to a dozen cherries a day in addition to drinking a glass of cherry juice. Find a happy medium by using your own good judgment as to cherry dosage. Listen to your body. You'll know soon enough if the cherries seem to be making you feel better.

Eat a portion of fresh string beans every day, or juice the string beans and drink a glassful daily. String beans contain vitamins A, B-1, B-2 and C and supposedly help over-acid conditions such as arthritis.

Steep 1 cup of fully packed parsley in 1 quart of boiling water. After 15 minutes, strain and refrigerate.

DOSE: ½ cup before breakfast, ½ cup before dinner and ½ cup anytime pain is particularly severe.

Garlic has been used to quiet arthritis pain quickly. Rub a freshly cut clove of garlic on painful areas. Also, take 2 garlic pills a day—after breakfast and after dinner.

Grate 3 tablespoonsful of horseradish and stir it into ½ cup of boiled milk. Pour the mixture onto a piece of cheesecloth, then apply it to the painful area. By the time the poultice cools, you may have some relief.

Celery contains many nourishing salts and organic sulphur. Some modern herbalists believe that celery has the power to help neutralize uric acid and other excess acids in the body. Eat fresh celery daily. The leaves on top of celery stalks are also good to eat. If the roughage is rough on your digestive system, place the tops and tough parts of the stalk in a non-aluminum pan. Cover with water and slowly bring to a boil. Then simmer for 10 to 15 minutes. Strain and pour into a jar.

DOSE: Drink 8 ounces 3 times a day, ½ hour before each meal.

You can vary your celery intake by drinking celery seed tea and/or juiced celery stalks, or do as the Rumanians do and cook celery in milk. Remember, celery is a diuretic, so plan your day accordingly.

According to results published in *The Journal of the American Medical Association*, based on experiments by a study team at the Brusch Medical Center in Massachusetts, cod-liver oil in milk helped to reduce cholesterol levels, improve blood chemistry and complexion, increase energy, and correct stomach problems, blood sugar balance, blood pressure and tissue inflammation.

Mix 1 tablespoonful of cod-liver oil (emulsified Norwegian cod-liver oil is non-fishy) in 6 ounces of milk.

DOSE: Drink it on an empty stomach, ½ hour before breakfast and ½ hour before dinner.

Applying cod-liver oil externally is said to help relieve the popping noises of the joints.

Even if you have a sensitivity to nightshade foods, external potato remedies can be used, as they have been for centuries. Carry a raw potato in your pocket. Don't leave home without it! When it shrivels up after a day or two, replace it with a fresh potato. It supposedly draws out the poisons and acids that might be causing the problem and pain.

For dealing with the affected areas more directly, dice 2 cups of unpeeled potatoes and put them in a non-aluminum saucepan with 5 cups of water. Boil gently until about half the water is left. While the water is hot, but not scalding, dunk a clean cloth in the potato water, wring it out and apply it to the painful parts of the body. Repeat the procedure for as long as your patience holds out, or the pain persists—whichever goes first.

When you're feeling twinges in the hinges all over your body, take a bath in rose petals. Use petals from 3 or 4 roses that are about to wither and throw them in your bath water. It should give you a rosy outlook.

Temporary Relief For Women Only: Arthritic pains often disappear when a woman is pregnant. As soon as researchers find the reason for this, they may also find a permanent cure.

Eating strawberries and very little else for a few days is said to be a possible cure for gout. Strawberries are a powerful alkalizer and contain calcium, iron and an ingredient known as salacin, which soothes inflammatory conditions. It worked so well for botanist Linnaeus that he referred to strawberries as "a blessing of the gods."

Apple cider vinegar has been used in various ways to help arthritis sufferers. See which remedy is most palatable and convenient for you. Don't forget to have patience and give it at least 3 weeks to work.

Every morning and every evening, take 1 teaspoonful of honey mixed with 1 teaspoonful of apple cider vinegar. Or: Before each meal (3 times a day), drink a glass of water containing 2 teaspoonsful of apple cider vinegar. Or: Between lunch and dinner, drink a mixture of 2 ounces of apple cider vinegar added to 6 ounces of water. Drink it down slowly.

Put an ounce of alfalfa seeds in ½ quart of hot, but not boiling, water and simmer for 30 minutes. Strain, cool and refrigerate it. DO NOT LET IT STAY IN THE REFRIGERATOR MORE THAN 24 HOURS. Sweeten to taste with honey. Drink the alfalfa tea at least 4 times a day—more if you possibly can. Once you feel all better, you can reduce your intake of the tea to 2 or 3 times a week.

Prepare a poultice of coarse (kosher) salt that has been heated in a frying pan. Then apply it to the painful area. To keep the salt comfortably warm, put a hot water bottle on top of it. (I'm sure this old home remedy draws out the pain effectively with non-kosher salt, too.)

‡ CHARLEY HORSE (MUSCLE STIFFNESS)

Prepare strong ginger tea with 2 teaspoonsful of ginger powder or fresh, grated ginger root in 2 cups of water. Let it simmer until the water turns yellow-ish in color. Add the ginger tea to a bathful of warm water. Relax in the tub for 20 to 30 minutes. This ginger tea bath may relieve muscle stiffness and soreness and is wonderful for one's circulation.

Soak in a tub of "old faithful"—Epsom salt. Pour 3 cupsful of it in warm water. Stay in the water 20 to 30 minutes and your charley horse pain may start to ease.

‡ SPRAINS

During the first 12 hours after the injury, starting as soon as possible, apply an ice-cold water compress to the area to reduce the swelling caused by the sprain. Leave the ice pack on for 20 minutes, then take it off for 20 minutes. Extend the 12 hours of cold compresses to 24 hours if necessary. It would be wise to seek medical attention to make sure the sprain is nothing more than a sprain and not a fractured, chipped or dislocated bone.

To help relieve the pain from a severe sprain, rub on leek liniment. To prepare the liniment, simmer 4 leeks in boiling water until they're mushy. Pour off the water and mash 4 tablespoonsful of coconut butter into the leek. As soon as it's cool, massage it into the sprained area. Keep the remaining liniment in a covered container. It can also be used for most muscle aches and pains.

‡Asthma

During an asthma attack, bronchial tubes narrow and secrete an excess of mucus, making it very hard to breathe.

Asthma in certain people may be attributed to allergies or emotional problems, or possibly a combination of both.

In the 1800s, Peter Latham said, "You cannot be sure of the success of your remedy, while you are still uncertain of the nature of the disease." And so it is with asthma.

Folk medicine legends abound with curious asthma remedies from around the world:

European and Australian folklore advocates swallowing a handful of spiderwebs rolled into a ball. Deep in the heart of Texas, they are said to sleep on the uncleaned wool of recently sheared sheep. The asthma is, legend has it, absorbed by the wool. Another old Texas home remedy requires the asthmatic to get a chihuahua (Mexican hairless dog). The theory is that the asthma goes from the patient to the dog, but the dog does not suffer from it. According to the folk of Kentucky, wearing a string of amber beads around the neck may cure asthma. With the cost of a full strand of amber these days, it would be cheaper to buy a chihuahua, have him get asthma, then buy that tiny dog a strand of amber.

These legendary folk remedies make for good conversation, but in the midst of an asthma attack, who can talk?

The remedies we recommend for asthmatic conditions are more practical and easier to come by than those listed above.

While trying to find the most effective asthma-relieving remedy, it's important that you consult with a health professional every step of the way. These remedies are not substitutions for professional medical treatment.

Eat 3 to 6 apricots a day. They may help promote healing of lung and bronchial conditions.

Jerusalem artichokes, eaten daily, may be a real plus for nourishing the lungs of the asthmatic. (See "Diabetes" for more details on these terrific tubers.)

Put 4 cups of sunflower seeds in 2 quarts of water and boil it down to 1 quart of water. Strain out the little pieces of sunflower seeds, then add 1 pint of honey and boil it down to a syrupy consistency.
DOSE: 1 teaspoonful ½ hour after each meal.

A relative told us that in the "old country," a remedy used at the onset of an asthma attack was to inhale the steam from boiling potatoes that were cut in pieces with the skin left on them. With or without the potatoes, inhaling steam can be beneficial. Be careful: Steam is powerful and can burn the skin.

Mix 1 teaspoonful of grated horseradish with 1 teaspoonful of honey and take it every night before bedtime.
Slice 2 large raw onions into a jar. Pour 2 cups of honey over it. Close the jar and let it stand overnight. Next morning you're ready to start taking the "honion" syrup.
DOSE: 1 teaspoonful ½ hour after each meal and 1 teaspoonful before bed.

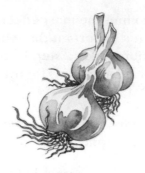

Similar to, but more potent than, the sunflower seed syrup described earlier in this chapter, is this garlic syrup. Separate and peel the cloves of 3 entire garlic bulbs. Simmer them in a non-aluminum pan with 2 cups of water. When the garlic cloves are soft and there's about a cup of water left in the pan, remove the garlic and put it in a jar. Then, add 1 cup of cider vinegar and ¼ cup of honey to the water that's left in the pan, boiling the mixture until it's syrupy. Pour the syrup over the garlic in the jar. Cover the jar and let it stand overnight.

DOSE: 1 or 2 cloves of garlic with a spoonful of syrup every morning on an empty stomach.

Buy either concentrated cranberry juice, sold at health food stores, or unconcentrated cranberry juice, sold at most supermarkets (READ THE IN-GREDIENTS ON THE LABEL and make sure there are no preservatives or sugar added), or make your own with 1 pound of cranberries in 1 pint of water. Boil until the cranberries are very mushy. Then, pour the mixture into a jar and keep it in the refrigerator.

DOSE: Drink 2 tablespoonsful ½ hour before each meal and at the onset of an asthma attack.

‡Blood

Blood is an extremely complex substance consisting of many liquid and solid elements including red and white blood cells, blood platelets and blood plasma.

The average adult has between 5 and 6 quarts of blood circulating through the body by way of the blood vessels.

To help circulation as well as purification of the blood and aid in elimination of iron-deficiency anemia, we offer suggestions *with* the suggestion you *first* have appropriate professional blood tests and consult with a physician *before* embarking on any self-help program.

‡ IRON-DEFICIENCY ANEMIA

Grape juice (no sugar or preservatives added), is a wonderful source of iron. Drink 8 ounces every day.

Eat raw spinach salads often. Be sure to wash the spinach thoroughly. Combine any of the following in your spinach salad: watercress, radish, kohlrabi, garlic, chives, leek and onion. they're all high in iron.

Every morning after breakfast and every evening after dinner, eat 2 dried apricots.

Snack on raisins.

NOTE: In the case of a serious iron deficiency, you may require more iron than you can possibly get from any or all of the suggestions above. We suggest you seek help from a health professional.

‡ BLOOD FORTIFIERS

Raw (not canned) sauerkraut is said to do a super job of fortifying the blood. It also helps rejuvenate the body in other ways. Eat 2 to 4 tablespoonsful a day, right after a meal. (See "Preparation Guide" and learn to prepare your own sauerkraut.)

CHECK WITH YOUR MEDICAL ADVISER BE-FORE GOING ON THIS 1-DAY FAST. Combine 2 tablespoonsful of lemon, 1 tablespoonful of honey and a cup of warm water.

DOSE: Every 2 hours, from morning until 2 hours before bedtime, take 2 tablespoonsful of the mixture. No food throughout the day, just the lemon/honey/water mixture.

Raw (not cooked or canned) pumpkin pulp and squash are said to have purifying properties. Eat them in salads.

When they're in season, a peach a day helps wash toxins away.

Garlic is said to help thin and fortify the blood. Eat raw garlic and/or take 2 garlic capsules daily.

Drink fresh carrot juice as often as once a day if you have access to a juicer, or eat raw carrots. They contain calcium, potassium, phosphorus, and vitamins A, B-1, B-2 and C.

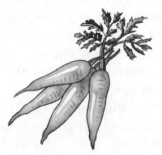

‡ CIRCULATION

Once a day, mix ⅛ teaspoonful of cayenne pepper in a cup of water and drink it down. It's not easy to take, but it may be beneficial to the circulatory system, since cayenne pepper is reputed to be the purest stimulant of all herbs.

Japanese medicine recommends ginger foot-baths to improve circulation. Add a cup of fresh, minced ginger to a basin with 2 quarts of warm water. Soak your feet in the water until they're rosy red. Then, dry thoroughly and notice a more energized feeling.

‡ VARICOSE VEINS

Reduce the swelling and constriction of varicose veins by wrapping a cheesecloth bandage soaked in witch hazel around the affected area. Lie down, raise your legs and relax.

At the end of every day, stand in a tub of cold water up to the knees. After 2 or 3 minutes, dry the legs with a coarse towel, then walk around your home at a brisk pace, also for about 2 to 3 minutes.

‡Blood Pressure

When blood pressure is measured, there are two numbers reported: the first and higher number is the systolic. It measures the pressure inside the arteries the second the heart beats. The diastolic is the lower number and measures the pressure in the arteries when the heart is at rest.

More than 20 million Americans have high blood pressure (hypertension). If you're one of those people, you are not alone.

You probably already know the following basics. Hopefully, you'll take a look at your life-style and, once and for all, do something about it!

- If you're overweight, diet sensibly (without diet pills). Eliminate salt and cut down or cut out meat.
- To reduce the stress from your everyday life, try biofeedback and/or meditation. Ask a health professional for guidance and reputable contacts.
- If you smoke, stop!
- If you drink, stop! or at least cut down drastically.

Read on for additional high and low blood pressure health hints.

‡ HIGH BLOOD PRESSURE

Eat 2 apples a day. The pectin in apples may help lower high blood pressure.

Eat raw garlic in salads and use it in cooking. Also take 2 garlic pills daily—1 after breakfast and 1 after dinner.

According to a university study, blood pressure can be reduced by staring at fish in a fish tank. The relaxation benefits of fish-watching are equal to biofeedback and meditation.

Cucumbers are rich in potassium, phosphorous and calcium. They're also a good diuretic and calming agent. To help bring down blood pressure, try eating a cucumber every day. If you have a juicer, drink ½ cup of fresh cucumber juice. You can also include some carrots and parsley in the juice.

First scrub, then boil unpeeled potatoes for 15 minutes. Let the potato water cool and drink 2 cups of it a day.

‡ BLOOD PRESSURE STABILIZERS

Just as there are people with high blood pressure, there are people (not as many) with low blood pressure. The following remedies are said to be blood pressure regulators and stabilizers:

Eat alfalfa sprouts daily. Save money by growing your own sprouts. (See "Preparation Guide" for sprouting instructions.) You may also want to supplement your sprout intake with 3 or 4 alfalfa tablets a day. Alfalfa is said to help fortify the blood, build resistance to disease and strengthen blood cells and arteries.

Scientific studies have shown that 5 to 10 minutes of laughter first thing in the morning improves blood pressure levels. The problem is, what's there to laugh at first thing in the morning? There may be a Dial-A-Joke in your area. (Check with your local information operator.) There's usually a funny local disc jockey on radio. Ask friends for recommendations, which should give you some laughs right there.

Eat raw garlic in salads and use it in cooking. Also take 2 garlic pills daily—1 after breakfast and 1 after dinner.

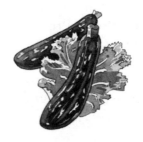

‡Burns

Burns are classified by degrees. A first-degree burn involves painful, red, unbroken skin. A second-degree burn involves painful blisters and broken skin. A third-degree burn destroys underlying tissue as well as surface skin. It may be painless because nerve endings may have also been destroyed. A fourth-degree burn involves deeply charred and blackened areas of the skin.

Second-degree burns that cover an extensive area of skin and *all* third- and fourth-degree burns require immediate medical attention. Any kind of burn on the face should also receive immediate medical attention as a precaution against swollen breathing passages.

As for first-degree burns—grabbing a hot pot handle, grasping the iron side of an iron, the oven door closing on your forearm, a splattering of boiling oil—here are first-aid suggestions for these burns, using mostly handy household items, that is, with the exception of cow dung and mud. Then again, if you're "home on the range," those *are* the handy household items.

‡ FIRST-DEGREE BURNS
Apply cold water or cold compresses first! Then—

Draw out the heat and pain by applying a slice of raw, unpeeled potato, or a piece of fresh pumpkin pulp, or a slice of raw onion. Leave the potato, pumpkin or onion on the burn for 15 minutes, off for

5 minutes and then put a fresh piece on for another 15 minutes.

If you burn yourself while baking and happen to have salt-free unbaked pie crust around, roll it thin and place it on the entire surface of the burn. Let it stay on until it dries up and falls off by itself.

If you have vitamin E or garlic oil capsules, puncture either one of them and squeeze the contents directly on the burn.

Uncooked chicken fat placed directly on burns and scalds is said to be quite soothing.

If you have a smooth piece of charcoal, put it on the burn and keep it there for an hour. Within minutes, the pain may begin to subside.

Make a poultice of raw sauerkraut and apply it to the burned area. If you don't have sauerkraut, use crushed comfrey root with a little honey. In fact, just plain honey on the burn may ease the pain and help the healing process.

If you're outdoors, pack mud on the burn to draw out the heat.

Spread apple butter over the burned area. As it dries, add another coat to it. Keep adding coats for a day or two, until the burn is just about butter—uh, better.

People have had remarkable results with apple cider vinegar. Pour it on the burned or scalded area.

Keep an aloe vera plant in your home. It's like growing a tube of ointment. Break off about a ½-inch piece of stem. Squeeze it so that the juice oozes out onto the burned area. The juice is most effective if the plant is at least two to three years old and the stems have little bumps on the edges.

‡ SECOND-DEGREE BURNS

For *at least* ½ hour, dip the burned area in cold water, or apply a towel that's been drenched in ice-cold water. DO NOT USE LARD, BUTTER OR A SALVE ON THE BURN! They seal in the heat, and when you get medical attention, the doctor has to wipe off the goo to see the condition of the skin.

If the burn is on an arm or leg, keep the limb raised in the air to help prevent swelling.

‡ CHEMICAL AND ACID BURNS

Until you get medical attention, immediately get the affected area under the closest running water—a sink, a garden hose, or the shower. The running water will help wash the chemicals off the skin. Keep the water running on the burned skin for at least 20 minutes or until medical help arrives.

‡ BURNED TONGUE

Keep rinsing mouth with cold water. A few drops of vanilla extract may relieve the pain.

‡ SUNBURN

When you've gotten more than you've basked for, fill a quart jar with equal parts of milk and ice and 2 tablespoonsful of salt. Soak a washcloth in the mixture and place it on the sunburned area. Leave it on for about 15 minutes. Repeat the procedure 3 to 4 times throughout the day.

Steep 6 regular (non-herbal) tea bags in a quart of hot water. When the tea is strong and cool, drench a washcloth in the liquid and apply it to the sunburned area. Repeat the procedure until you get relief.

Spread yogurt or sour cream over the sunburned area, particularly the face. Leave it on for 20 minutes, then rinse off with lukewarm water. The yogurt or sour cream is said to take the heat out of the sunburn and tighten pores, too.

NOTE: Severe sunburns can be second-degree burns. If sunburned skin is broken or blistering, treatment should include cold water followed by a dry (preferably sterile) dressing.

‡ SUNBURNED EYES

Make a poultice of grated apples and rest it on your closed eyelids for a relaxing hour.

Make a poultice from the lightly beaten white of an egg. Bandage the poultice on the closed eyes and leave it there overnight. There may be a big improvement next morning.

‡Colds, Etc.

If you're out there with a red, runny nose, chest congestion and that achy flu feeling, instead of making much achoo about nothing, keep reading for some simple cold-helping hints.

‡ COLDS/FLU

The first round of ammunition for fighting the cold war is Chicken Soup (Jewish penicillin). According to *Medical World News*, July 10, 1978, the director of medical services at Mount Sinai Medical Center in Miami Beach, Dr. Marvin A. Sackner, proved that chicken soup can help cure a cold.

Using a bronchofiberscope and cineroentgenograms and measurements of mucus velocity, Dr. Sackner tested the effectiveness of hot chicken soup and hot and cold water. Cold water lowered nasal clearance. Hot water improved it, but it was nothing compared to the improvement after hot chicken soup. Then, to negate the effects of the steam from the hot water and hot chicken soup, the fluids were sipped through straws from covered containers. Hot water had very little effect this way. The hot chicken soup still had some benefit.

CHICKEN SOUP RECIPE:

- 4–5 pounds of chicken parts
- 3 carrots, scrubbed or peeled, cut in thirds
- 2 parsnips, scrubbed, cut in thirds
- 2 celery stalks with leaves, cut in thirds
- 1 large onion cut in half
- 1 green pepper, cut in half and cleaned out
- 2 sprigs dill (optional), or ½ teaspoonful of dill seeds
- 4 parsley sprigs
- 4 cloves of garlic, crushed
- 1 to 2 teaspoonsful of salt
- 10 cups of water

Add the chicken, carrots, parsnips, celery, onion, green pepper, water and salt to a big pot. Wrap the dill or dill seeds, parsley and garlic in cheesecloth and add that to the pot. Bring it to a boil, clean off the scum from the top of the soup, cover and simmer for 2½ to 3 hours. If, after 3 hours, the soup is lacking the flavor you want, add a few chicken boullion cubes to taste. Remove the chicken and the vegetables. Refrigerate the soup overnight. Next day, before heating the soup, remove the top layer of fat, skimming the surface with a spoon. Add the vegetables, heat and—Eat! Eat! Before it gets cold!

In the USSR, garlic is known as Russian penicillin. It has been reported that colds have actually disappeared within hours—a day at most—after taking garlic. Keep a peeled clove of garlic in the mouth, between the cheek and teeth. Do not chew it. Occasionally, release a little garlic juice by digging the teeth into the clove. Replace the clove every 3 to 4 hours.

Combine a crushed clove of garlic with ½ tea-spoonful of cayenne pepper, the juice of 1 lemon, 1,000 mg of vitamin C (buy it powdered or grind it yourself), and 1 teaspoonful of honey.

DOSE: Take mixture 3 times a day at mealtime.

If taking garlic by mouth is not for you, then peel and crush 6 cloves of garlic. Mix them into ½ cup of white lard. Spread the mush on the soles of the feet and cover them with a (preferably warmed) towel or flannel cloth. Put paper toweling under the feet to absorb grease. Garlic is so powerful that even though it's applied to one's feet, it will be on one's breath, too.

DOSE: Apply a fresh batch of garlic and lard every 5 hours until the cold is gone.

Prepare tea by steeping equal parts of cinnamon, sage and bay leaves in hot water. Before drinking the tea, add 1 tablespoonful of lemon juice.

Keep flushing out your system by drinking lots of non-dairy liquids—unsweetened fruit juices, herbal tea (see above) and just plain water.

When our friend, the contessa from the Italian hills, has a cold, she makes a mug of very strong, regular tea and adds 1 tablespoonful of honey, 1 tablespoonful of cognac, 1 teaspoonful of butter and ¼ teaspoonful of cinnamon. She drinks it as hot as she can and goes to bed between cotton sheets. If she wakes up during the night and is all sweaty, she changes her bedclothes and sheets and goes back to bed. By morning, she feels *"molto bene!"*

People have been known to fake a cold just to take this: Combine 4 teaspoonsful of rum with the juice of 1 lemon and 3 teaspoonsful of honey. Then add it to a glass of hot water and drink it before retiring. And don't tell us you plan to retire in another 14 years.

Mix ¼ cup of apple cider vinegar with an equal amount of honey. It's an elixir that is particularly effective for a cold with a sore throat.

DOSE: Take 1 tablespoonful 6 to 8 times a day.

Boil down ½ cup of sunflower seeds (without the shells, of course) in 5 cups of water until there's about 2 cups of liquid left in the pot. Then stir in ¼ cup of honey and ¾ cup of gin. This potion is particularly good for chest colds.

DOSE: Take 2 teaspoonsful 3 times a day at mealtime.

Mix the white of 1 raw egg with 4 teaspoonsful of prepared mustard and rub it on the chest. Take a (preferably white) towel and dip it in hot water, then wring it out and place it on top of the mixture already on the chest. As soon as the towel is cool, redip it in hot water, wring it out and again, put it back on the chest. Reapply the towel 4 or 5 times. After the last application of the towel, wash off the chest, dry thoroughly, bundle up and go to bed.

To stimulate appropriate acupuncture points that can help a cold, place an ice cube on the bottom of both big toes. Keep them in place with an Ace bandage or piece of cloth. Place feet in a basin or on plastic to avoid a mess from the melting ice. Do this procedure morning, noon and night.

In *Atlantic* magazine, a doctor wrote this cold remedy that we do NOT recommend: "To treat the common cold, go to bed with a bottle of whiskey and a hat. Place hat on left-hand bedpost. Take a drink of whiskey and move hat to right-hand bedpost. Take another drink and shift it back again. Continue until you drink the whiskey but fail to move the hat. By then the cold is probably cured."

‡ **FEVER**

Bind sliced onions or peeled garlic cloves to the bottoms of the feet. Don't be surprised if it gives you onion or garlic breath. And, don't be surprised if it brings down your temperature.

Eat grapes (in season) throughout the day. Also, dilute pure grape juice and sip some of it throughout the day. Drink it at room temperature, never chilled.

Boil 4 cups (1 quart) of water with ½ teaspoonful of cayenne pepper. As you're ready to drink each of these 4 cups throughout the day, add to each cup 1 teaspoonful of honey and ¼ cup of orange juice. Heat it up just a little and then drink it slowly.

‡ **SINUS**

Slowly, cautiously and gently inhale the vapors of freshly grated horseradish (known in certain circles as the Jewish Dristan). While you're at it, mix grated horseradish with lemon juice (equal amounts of each).

DOSE: Eat 1 teaspoonful 1 full hour before breakfast and at least 1 hour after dinner. It gives long-lasting relief to some sinus sufferers who are good about taking it every day without fail.

Crush 1 clove of garlic into ¼ cup of water. Sip up the garlicky water into an eyedropper. (Make sure no pieces get into the dropper.)

DOSE: 10 drops of clear garlic water per nostril, 3 times a day for 3 days. At the end of the 3 days, there should be a noticeable clearing up of the sinus infection.

Buy garlic pills and parsley pills.

DOSE: Take 2 garlic pills and 2 parsley pills every 4 hours that you're awake. (That should add up to 4 times a day.) At the end of 6 days, you should be breathing a lot easier.

To stop sniffling, swallow 1 teaspoonful of honey with freshly ground pepper sprinkled on it. Don't inhale the pepper or you'll get rid of the sniffles and start sneezing.

‡ HAY FEVER

Chew a bite-size chunk of honeycomb at the start of a hay fever attack. The honey is delicious. The comb part turns into a ball of wax that should be chewed for 10 to 15 minutes. Our experience has been that it gives temporary relief from a hay fever attack.

The U.S. Army tested honeycomb as a desensitizing and anti-allergic substance for hay fever. Their results were very encouraging, especially those from patients who chewed the honeycomb. (After chewing the waxy stuff, throw it out rather than swallow it.)

(See "And Now May We Prevent..." for immunizing against hay fever.)

Several studies have shown that bioflavonoids help the body utilize vitamin C more effectively.

After the morning and evening meals, take 1 pantothenic acid (50 mg) and 1 vitamin C (500 mg) tablet along with a bioflavonoid—a grapefruit, orange, a few strawberries, grapes or prunes. If you don't want a fruit, take a teaspoonful of grated orange or lemon peel sweetened with a little honey. This remedy has been said to have brought relief to many hay fever sufferers.

‡ NOSEBLEEDS

Always keep your head elevated. Do not lie down.

NOTE: Nasal hemorrhaging—blood flowing from both nostrils—requires immediate medical attention. Rush to the nearest doctor or hospital emergency room.

Recurrent nosebleeds may be a symptom of an underlying ailment. Seek appropriate medical attention.

When one of us had a nosebleed, our father would take a half-dollar, put it on the frozen ice cube tray for a few seconds, then press it to the back of the sufferer's neck. We looked forward to getting nosebleeds, since we would get to keep the half-dollar.

Ice at the nape of the neck has also been known to work, as has raw onion, but neither is as profitable.

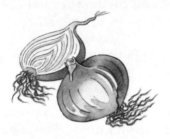

Nosebleeds have been known to stop when you immerse your hands in warm water. Well, that's something to be said for doing the dishes: You'll never get a nosebleed while doing them.

Take your thumb and forefinger and pinch your nose right below the hard, bony part—about halfway down the nose. Stay that way for 7 minutes, and you should no longer have a nosebleed.

Fold a small piece of brown paper and place it between the upper lip and the gum. It's been known to stop a bloody nose in no time.

‡Constipation and Regularity

You are most likely reading this page because you're seeking a natural laxative. Therefore, you may already know that the commercial chemical laxatives can kill friendly bacteria, can lessen the absorption of nutrients, can stuff up the intestinal walls, can turn users into addicts, can get rid of necessary vitamins and can eventually *cause* constipation.

We offer easy-to-take, inexpensive, non-chemical constipation relievers that should not present any problem side effects if taken in moderation, using good common sense. In other words, don't try more than one remedy at a time.

NOTE: Constipation is a common problem that may be a symptom of disease or lead to more major health problems. It is important to consult with your medical authority before starting any self-help treatment.

‡ CONSTIPATION

The most natural time to move your bowels is within the first few hours of the day. Drinking water on an empty stomach stimulates peristalis by reflex. So, before breakfast, drink the juice of ½ lemon in 1 cup of warm water. It may help cleanse your system and make you pucker a lot. If you find it hard to drink, sweeten it with honey.

Instead of lemon in water, eat or drink any of the following at room temperature (not chilled):

- Prune juice or stewed prunes
- Papaya
- 2 peeled apples
- 6 to 8 dried figs. Soak them overnight in a glass of water. In the morning, drink the water, then eat the figs.
Have only one kind of fruit for breakfast and do not overdo the portion.

The combination of dried apricots and prunes is said to work wonders. Soak 6 of each overnight. Next morning, eat 3 of each. Then, in the late afternoon, an hour or two before dinner, eat the remaining 3 apricots and 3 prunes.

We have tried to stay away from commercial products, but this one works so well, we must share it with you. It's Uncle Sam's Cereal with Flaxseed. While you're at the health food store buying the cereal, pick up a bag of flaxseed and add an extra tablespoonful to the cereal each morning. You'll pledge allegiance to Uncle Sam's because of the results. Incidentally, some supermarkets also stock the cereal.

If you insist on your favorite brand of cereal, add raw, unprocessed bran to it. Start with 1 teaspoonful and gradually work your way up to 1 or 2 tablespoonsful each morning, depending on your reaction to it.

Here are two natural laxatives available at your green grocer: escarole (eat it raw or boil it in water and drink the water), and Spanish onion (roast it and eat it at bedtime). The cellulose in onions gives intestinal momentum.

Raw sauerkraut and its juice have friendly bacteria and may aid digestion. It's also an excellent laxative. Heat destroys the important enzymes in sauerkraut, so make sure you eat it raw. (See "Preparation Guide" and learn to prepare your own sauerkraut.)

You can also drink the sauerkraut juice to help you overcome constipation. Combine ⅓ of a glass of kraut juice with ⅔ of a glass of tomato juice and drink it down slowly.

Hippocrates, the Father of Medicine, recommended eating garlic every day to relieve constipation. Cook with it and eat it raw (in salads) whenever possible.

Just as you're falling asleep, when the mind is most open to autohypnotic suggestion, say to yourself, "In the morning, I will have a good bowel movement." Keep repeating the sentence until you doze off. Pleasant dreams!

‡ MILD LAXATIVES
Raw spinach makes a delicious salad, has lots of vitamins and minerals and is a mild laxative, too.

One teaspoonful of blackstrap molasses in ½ cup of warm water an hour before lunch might do the trick.

Soak your feet in cold water, 15 minutes at a time, once in the morning and once before bedtime. Be sure to dry the feet thoroughly.

Okra acts as a mild laxative. Add chicken gumbo soup to your menu from time to time. Here's a recipe that will give you 6 delicious servings:

CHICKEN GUMBO SOUP WITH OKRA
- 1 small, cleaned chicken cut into serving portions
- 2 tablespoonsful of flour
- 1 onion, chopped
- 2 tablespoonsful of vegetable oil
- 4 cups of okra, chopped
- 2 cups of tomato pulp
- ¼ cup of parsley, chopped
- 4 cups water
- Salt and pepper

Coat chicken pieces lightly with flour and sauté with onion in oil. Add okra, tomato, parsley and water as soon as chicken is browned. Season with salt and pepper to taste. Simmer for about 2½ hours, until chicken is tender and okra is well cooked. Be sure to add water as needed during the 2½ hours of simmering.

‡ STOOL SOFTENER

Every night, before eating dinner, eat a tablespoonful of raisins or 3 prunes that have been soaking in water for a couple of hours.

‡Coughs

In the morning, when the doctor examined her patient, she remarked, "I'm happy to say your cough sounds much better."

The patient answered, "Well, it should. I had a whole night of practice."

We all have a cough center in our brain. It's generally motivated by an irritation in the respiratory tract. In other words, a cough is nature's way of helping us loosen and get rid of mucus that's congesting our system.

Here are some folk remedies that may bring back memories of when you were a child and had a cough.

NOTE: If cough persists, have it checked by a health professional.

‡ COUGHS IN GENERAL

For 5 minutes, cook the juice of 1 lemon, 1 cup of honey and ½ cup olive oil. Then stir vigorously for a couple of minutes.

DOSE: 1 teaspoonful every 2 hours.

Combine ½ cup apple cider vinegar with ½ cup water. Add 1 teaspoonful of cayenne pepper and sweeten to taste with honey.

DOSE: 1 tablespoonful when the cough starts acting up. Another tablespoonful at bedtime.

Peel and finely chop 6 medium onions. Put them and ½ cup of honey into the top of a double boiler, or in a pan over a pot of boiling water. Cover the mixture and let it simmer for 2 hours. Strain this concoction we call "honion," and pour it into a jar with a cover.

DOSE: 1 warm tablespoonful every 2 to 3 hours.

Grate 1 teaspoonful of horseradish and mix it with 2 teaspoonsful of honey. (1 finely chopped clove of garlic can be used in place of horseradish.)

DOSE: 1 teaspoonful every 2 to 3 hours.

For a delicious, thirst-quenching and soothing drink, squeeze the juice of 1 lemon into a big mug or glass. Add hot water, 2 tablespoonsful of honey and either 3 whole cloves, or ½-inch piece of stick cinnamon.

DOSE: 1 glassful every 3 hours.

Cook a cup of barley according to the directions on the package. Add the juice of 1 fresh lemon and some water to the cooked barley. Then, liquefy the mixture in a blender. Drink it slowly.

DOSE: 1 cup every 4 hours.

Cut a hole through the middle of a rutabaga or a yellow onion and fill the hole with honey or brown sugar. Leave it overnight. In the morning, drink the juice and it will relieve the cough.

Cut a deep hole in the middle of a large beet and fill the hole with honey or brown sugar. Bake the beet until it's soft. It's a treat to eat the beet... whenever you feel a cough coming on.

Adding spices and herbs to wine is called mulling. You might want to mull this over for your cough.

Into 3 cups of wine, add a 1-inch piece of stick cinnamon, 1 tablespoonful of honey, 3 to 6 cloves (depending on how much you like the taste of cloves) and a few pieces of well-scrubbed lemon peel. Heat and stir.

DOSE: 3 cups a day.

Even if this mulled wine doesn't help, you somehow don't mind as much having the cough.

Chew on a bite-size piece of ginger root, just like you would chew gum. Swallowing the juice should help control a cough. Ginger is strong, and it might take some getting used to.

Take a piece of brown paper, about the size of your chest, and soak it in vinegar. When it stops dripping, sprinkle black pepper on one side of the paper. Then place the peppered side on your bare chest. To keep it in place overnight, wrap an Ace bandage or cloth around the chest. By morning, there may be a big improvement, particularly with a bronchial cough.

Among other ingredients, the polyunsaturated fatty acids in whole grain oats have been said to soothe bronchial inflammation and relieve coughing spasms.

Make a mash from the oats by following the directions on the whole grain oats box, but reduce the amount of water by ¼ cup. Add honey to taste.

DOSE: Eat 1 cup at a time, 4 times a day and whenever a coughing spell starts. Be sure the oat mash is eaten warm.

‡ DRY COUGH

Scrub 3 potatoes, then boil them with the skins on. Save the water and sweeten it with honey.

DOSE: 1 tablespoonful each time the cough acts up.

‡ NIGHT COUGH

To help loosen phlegm, fry 2 finely chopped medium onions in lard. As soon as it's cool enough to touch, rub the mixture on the cougher's chest and wrap the chest with a clean (preferably white) cloth. Do this procedure in the evening. It may give you a better night's sleep.

Right before bed, add 1 teaspoonful of dry mustard powder to a half-filled bathtub of hot water. Prepare a hot drink—take your choice: peppermint tea or hot water, honey and lemon. Wear bedclothes that leave the chest accessible. Have 2 rough terrycloth towels and a comfortable chair or stool in the bathroom. Dip your feet in water and keep them there for 15 minutes. (The rest of the body should be seated alongside the tub.) When the water cools, add more hot water. Sip the drink through this entire process. After 15 minutes of sipping and dipping (no stripping), dunk the towel in the bathwater, wring it out and place it on the bare chest. Once the towel cools off, dunk it again, wring it out and place it back on the chest. Repeat this 3 times, then dry the body thoroughly, bundle up and go to bed.

‡ NERVOUS COUGH

We know a stage manager who wants to make this announcement before the curtain goes up: "To stop nervous-type coughs, apply pressure to the area between your lip and your nose. If that doesn't work, press hard on the roof of the mouth. If neither works, please wait till intermission, then go outside and cough."

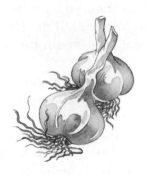

‡Depression, Nervousness and Fatigue

We all go through periods of depression, nervousness and fatigue. Maybe it's the weather—you know, a change of season. Or for women, it could be that time of month again. Of course, pressures at the office don't help, nor do tense relationships at work and at home. Then there are additives in foods and side effects from medications that can cause chemical imbalances that can lead to depression, nervousness and fatigue.

Whatever the reason, valid or not, when you're going through a bad time and you reach the point where you say to yourself, "I'm sick and tired of being sick and tired!" you're on the road to recovery.

If you are really ready to help yourself, you might start by cutting down on your sugar intake. Excessive sugar can help cause depression, nervous tension and spurts of energy followed by extreme fatigue. Caffeine products (coffee, non-herbal tea, cola, chocolate and some medications), cigarettes and alcoholic beverages may also contribute to nervous anxiety, depression and highs-and-lows of energy. Take them out of your life. They're taking the life out of you.

Eat a sensible diet of whole grains, steamed green vegetables, lean meat and fish, and raw garlic in big salads with sprouts, onion and lots of celery. Have sunflower seeds, raisins, sauerkraut, whole wheat pasta and beans. What could be bad?

For cases of deep depression, extreme nervousness and chronic fatigue, it may not be as simple as this. We suggest you seek professional assistance to help pinpoint the cause.

Some more anxiety-relieving recommendations are on the next few pages.

‡ DEPRESSION

Have a pizza with lots of oregano. If you don't have the oregano, forget the pizza. In fact, forget the pizza and just have the oregano. Oregano may ease that depressed, heavy-hearted feeling.

If you have a juicer, whip up half a glass of watercress and half a glass of spinach. Throw in some carrots to make the juice sweeter. Then, bottoms up and spirits up.

Eat 2 ripe bananas a day to chase the blues away. Bananas contain the chemicals serotonin and nor-epinephrine, which are believed to help prevent mental depression.

While running a warm bath, prepare a cup of camomile tea. Add the used teabag to the bath, along with a new one. If you use loose camomile, then wrap the herb in cheesecloth before putting it in the tub to avoid messy cleanup. Once the bath is ready, take pen and paper along with your cup of tea and relax in the tub. Make a list of a dozen wishes as you sip your tea. Be careful...the things you wish for may come true.

Cheer yourself up by wearing rose colors—pink and scarlets. The orange family of colors are also picker-uppers.

Making love can help people overcome feelings of depression—unless, of course, they have no one to make love to and that's why they're depressed.

‡ NERVOUS TENSION AND ANXIETY

Juices seem to be calming to the nerves. Throughout the day, sip apple, pineapple, prune, grape and cherry juice. While you're at it, add an egg yolk to the glass of cherry juice, stir and drink. Make sure the juices have no added sugar or preservatives, and drink them at room temperature, not chilled.

Chop a large onion into very small tidbits and add a tablespoonful of honey. Eat half the mixture with lunch and the other half with dinner. Onions contain prostaglandin, which is reported to have a tension-relieving effect.

If strawberries are in season, eat a few as a dessert after each meal (without the cream and sugar!). You may *feel* a difference (you won't be as edgy), and you may *see* a difference (they'll make your teeth whiter).

Peppermint tea has a wonderful way of relaxing the system and relieving moodiness. Drink it warm and strong.

If you are on edge, high-strung and, generally speaking, a nervous wreck, surround yourself with calming colors. Green has a harmonizing effect, since it's the color of nature. Earth colors should make you feel better. Wear quiet blues and gentle grays. It helps more than we realize.

Sage tea can help relieve the jitters. Steep a sage tea bag or 1 teaspoonful of sage in 1 cup of warm water for 5 minutes. Strain and drink 3 cups a day. A bonus: Sage tea also helps strengthen one's brain and memory.

There's a reason Epsom salts, an ancient natural healer, is still popular—it works! Pour 2 cups of Epsom salts into a warm-water bath. Set aside ½ hour for pure relaxation in the tub—no interruptions—just 30 minutes of tension-free fantasizing.

According to European folklore, celery helps you forget your troubles from a broken heart and soothes your nerves at the same time. Pass the celery, please.

‡ NERVOUS TICS
From time to time I get a tic around my eye. I feel like I'm winking at everyone. The tic-off switch that works like magic for me is 300 mg of vitamin B-6 a day.

‡ FATIGUE

If you're tired the second you awaken in the morning, try this Vermont tonic: In a blender, put 1 cup of warm water, 2 tablespoonsful of apple cider vinegar and 1 teaspoonful of honey. Blend thoroughly, then sip it slowly till it's all gone. Have this tonic every morning before breakfast, and within days, you may feel a difference in your energy level.

A quick picker-upper is ⅛ teaspoonful of cayenne pepper in a cup of water. Drink it down and get a second wind.

If you're suffering from mental fatigue, try this Austrian recipe: Thoroughly wash an apple, cut it into small pieces, leaving the peel on, and place the pieces in a bowl. Pour 2 cups of boiling water over the apple and let it steep for an hour. Then add 1 tablespoonful of honey. Drink the apple/honey water and eat the pieces of apple.

If possible, walk barefoot in dewy grass. Next best thing is to carefully walk up and back in 6 inches of cold bathwater. Do it from 5 to 10 minutes in the morning and late afternoon.

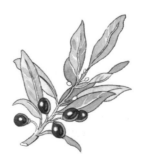

‡Diabetes

In simplified terms, diabetes is a condition in which the pancreas does not produce an adequate amount of insulin to burn up our intake of sugars and starches.

Many cases of diabetes can be completely controlled—controlled, not cured—by a sensible diet. By sticking to a low-calorie, high-carbohydrate diet with plenty of fiber, and exercising (walking at a normal speed for ½ hour after every meal), those diabetics remain drug-free and feel better than ever. The importance of controlled weight loss, especially for the obese, cannot be overemphasized.

Thanks to modern laboratory technology, diabetics can perform urinalysis and blood sugar tests conveniently in their own homes. While it makes it easy to monitor one's self, please remember:

DIABETES IS A SERIOUS CONDITION. DO NOT EMBARK ON ANY PLAN OF TREATMENT WITHOUT A DOCTOR'S SUPERVISION.

Along with a well-balanced, sugar-free diet, the combination of garlic, watercress and parsley, eaten daily, might help regulate the blood sugar level for some diabetics.

Sunchokes, also known as Jerusalem artichokes, although they're not from Jerusalem and they are not artichokes, eaten daily, have been said to help stimulate the production of insulin. They are tubers that contain inulin and levulin, carbohydrates that do not convert to sugar in the body. Jerusalem artichokes are similar in texture to potatoes, but they're sweeter-tasting. They're great for helping you stick to a reducing diet because they satisfy your sweet tooth, are low in calories and high in vitamins and minerals. Eat them raw as a snack or in salads, boiled in soups, or baked in stews.

Some green grocers are now carrying them. These tubers are easy to grow and worth the effort if you have the space. Ask your local nursery to help you get started.

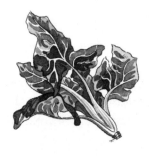

‡Diarrhea and Dysentery

Diarrhea is a common condition usually caused by overeating, or a minor bacterial infection, or mild food poisoning, and sometimes by emotional anxiety or extreme fatigue.

Even a quick and simple bout of diarrhea depletes the system of potassium and magnesium, often leaving the sufferer tired, depressed and dehydrated. It's important to keep drinking during and after a siege in order to avoid depletion and dehydration.

NOTE: If diarrhea persists, it may be a symptom of a more serious ailment. Get professional medical attention.

P.S.: "Diarrhea" pronounced backwards is "air raid."

‡ DIARRHEA

Since Biblical times, the common blackberry plant has been used to cure diarrhea and dysentery. And so the berry remedy, in one form or another, has been passed down through the generations. Don't be surprised if your neighborhood bartender recommends some blackberry brandy.

DOSE: 1 shot glass (2 tablespoonsful) every 4 hours.

Blackberry juice or wine will also do fine.

DOSE: 6 oz blackberry juice every 4 hours—or 2 oz (4 tablespoonsful) blackberry wine every 4 hours.

Scrape a peeled apple with a (preferably non-metal) spoon and eat it. In fact, eat no other food but grated apple until the condition greatly subsides.

If you're going on a honeymoon to Mexico, be sure to catch and save the rice that's thrown after the wedding. Boil ½ cup of (preferably brown) rice in 6 cups of water for ½ hour. Strain the water through cheesecloth, then sweeten the water with honey.

DOSE: Drink 1 cupful of the rice water every other hour. Do not drink other liquids until the condition disappears.

Eating cooked rice with a dash of cinnamon is also helpful in controlling the problem.

Bananas may help promote the growth of beneficial bacteria in the intestine and replace some of the lost potassium.

DOSE: 3 times a day, eat 1 ripe banana that has been soaked in milk.

Add 1 finely chopped teaspoonful of garlic to 1 teaspoonful of honey and swallow it down 3 times a day—2 hours after each meal.

Lactic acid drinks are effective in treating diarrhea and important in that they replenish the system's supply of friendly intestinal bacteria. Have 1 to 2 glasses of buttermilk or sauerkraut juice or kefir (found in health food stores). Or eat a portion or two of yogurt, pickled beets, pickled cucumbers or raw sauerkraut (see "Preparation Guide" for sauerkraut recipe).

‡ DYSENTERY

It is common for people traveling in foreign countries to get dysentery. All of the above remedies may help treat bacterial dysentery. However, amoebic dysentery (caused by amoeba living in the raw green vegetables of some countries) and viral dysentery are more severe forms of dysentery and should be treated by a health professional. (See "Dysentery" in "And Now May We Prevent...")

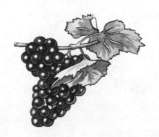

‡Ears

An earache is generally an infection of the middle ear, usually as a result of a cold or the flu. The pain can be out of proportion to the seriousness of the problem.

In the 1700s, satirist and physicist Georg Lichtenberg said, "What a blessing it would be if we could open and shut our ears as easily as we do our eyes."

If your ears are troubling you, keep your eyes open long enough to read the suggestions that follow.

NOTE: If an earache persists, don't turn a deaf ear! Check it out with a health professional.

‡ EARACHES

Puncture 1 garlic oil capsule and let the contents ooze into the ear. Gently plug the ear with a puff of cotton. The earache may ease considerably within a half-hour.

Combine 4 drops of onion juice with 1 teaspoonful of warm (not hot) olive oil.

DOSE: 3 drops in each ear in the morning (providing, of course, both ears ache) and 3 drops in each ear in the evening. Be sure to plug the ears with cotton puffs after applying the drops.

Mix ½ cup of unprocessed bran with ½ cup of coarse (kosher) salt and envelop it in a generous piece of folded-over cheesecloth. In other words, bundle it up so it doesn't spill all over the place. Then heat it in a low oven until it's warm but bearable to the touch. Place it on the painful ear for an hour.

Put castor oil on a piece of cotton. Sprinkle the oiled cotton with black pepper and apply it to the aching ear—not *in* the ear canal, *on* the ear.

If you're going to get an earache, try to get it when you're baking rye bread. All you have to do is take 1 ounce of caraway seeds and pummel them. Then add 1 cup of breadcrumbs from a soft, hot, newly baked loaf of bread and wrap it all in a piece of cheesecloth. Apply it to the sore ear. If you use already cooled bread, warm the poultice in the oven before applying it.

‡ INFLAMED EAR
Mix 1 tablespoonful of milk with 1 tablespoonful of olive oil or castor oil and heat.

DOSE: Put 4 drops of the mixture into the inflamed ear every hour and gently plug it up with cotton. Be sure the drops are not too hot.

‡ RUNNY, ABSCESSED EAR

Make a poultice of roasted onion and apply it to the infected ear. It should be as warm as can be without burning that tender, already infected area.

‡ GETTING THE BUGS OUT

It happens! Not often, but once in a blue moon, an insect will get inside a person's ear. Since insects are attracted to light, if an insect gets in your ear, turn toward the sun. Hopefully, the insect will fly out and away. If it occurs at night, shut the lights in the room and shine a flashlight in your ear. If it happens in a movie theatre, you're in luck. Just call the usher.

If the insect in your ear couldn't care less about the light, pour 1 teaspoonful of warm olive oil into your ear and hold it there a minute or two. Then tilt your head so that the oil and the bug come floating out. If that doesn't work, gently fill your ear with warm water. That should push out the insect and the oil.

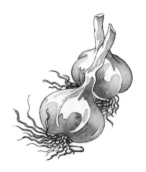

‡ RINGING

Ringing in the ears may be the result of a mild overdose of salycilate, which is found in aspirin, or other drugs. The ringing should stop when the drug is discontinued.

If you still hear ringing and there's no one there and you're not in love...Try onion juice.

DOSE: 2 drops of onion juice in your ears, 3 times a week should stop the ringing.

Believe it or not, a heating pad on your feet and one on your hands may ease the ringing in your ears. It all has to do with blood being redistributed, improving circulation and lessening pressure in congested areas.

NOTE: If ringing persists, it might be a sign of a more serious illness, in which case you should seek medical attention.

‡ GETTING THE WAX OUT

Sprinkle black pepper into 1 tablespoon of warm corn oil, then dip a puff of cotton into it and gently put the cotton into your ear. Remove the cotton in 5 minutes.

Warm 1 tablespoonful of hydrogen peroxide. Put 10 drops in the ear and let it fizz there for 3 minutes. Then tilt your head so that the liquid runs out onto a tissue. The wax should be softened. Gently remove the wax with soft cotton. Repeat the procedure with the other ear.

‡ BURNING EARS
Just tell people to stop talking about you!

‡ RESTORE AND/OR IMPROVE HEARING
Pinch the tip of your middle finger 4 times a day, 5 minutes each time. It's easy if you organize it this way: before every meal, pinch the right finger. After every meal, pinch the left finger. When you get up in the morning, pinch the right finger. When you go to bed at night, pinch the left finger.

Your right finger is for your right ear and left finger for left ear, so if you want to improve only one ear, pinch accordingly. Make it easy on yourself and clip on a clothespin.

This potent potion has been said to actually restore hearing: drink 1 ounce of garlic juice with 1 ounce of onion juice once a day. [See "Bad Breath" (Halitosis), immediately!]

Nothing improves a person's hearing like overhearing.

NOTE: You should seek professional medical attention for a hearing impairment or sudden hearing loss.

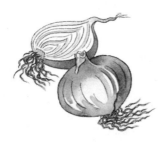

‡Eyes

How very precious our eyes and sight are to us. Agreed? Agreed! Then what have you done for your eyes lately? Do you know there's eye food, eye-strengthening exercises, an acupressure eyestrain reliever, eyewashes to brighten those baby blues, browns or greens, and natural healing alternatives to chemical symptom cover-ups?

There is an optometrist with a sign in his office window: "If you don't see what you want, you're in the right place."

Likewise. Read the following eye care suggestions, or get someone to read them to you.

‡ STIES

Place a handful of fresh parsley in a soup bowl. Pour a cup of boiling water over the parsley and let it steep for 10 minutes. Soak a clean washcloth in the hot water, lie down, put the cloth on your closed lid and relax for 15 minutes. Repeat the procedure before bedtime. Parsley water is also good for eliminating puffiness around the eyes.

Moisten a regular (non-herbal) tea bag, put it on the closed eye with the sty, bandage it in place and leave the bandage on overnight. Hopefully, by morning it will be bye-bye sty.

Rub the sty 3 times with a gold wedding ring. We decided not to use any silly-sounding, superstition-based remedies. In fact, we've discarded dozens of them, saving the lives of lots of toads, snakes and black cats. This remedy for sties, however, comes from so many reputable sources that it must have some credibility. Fortunately for us, but unfortunately for research purposes, neither of us has had a sty since working on this book, so we haven't been able to personally test the wedding-ring remedy. In the time you've spent reading all this, you could have rubbed the sty 3 times and written to tell us if it works. Could you please do that right now? Thanks. (Our mailing address is in the Introduction.)

‡ CINDERS

If you have something in your eye besides a contact lens, grasp your upper lid lashes firmly between your thumb and index finger. Gently pull the lashes toward the cheek, as far as you can without pulling them out. Hold it, count to 10, spit 3 times and let go of the lashes. Is it out? Repeat the procedure one more time. If it still doesn't work, get an onion and read the next remedy.

Mince an onion and let your tears wash away the cinder in your eye. It works every time.

‡ CHEMICALS

When chemicals like hair dye get in the eye, immediately wash the eye thoroughly with lots of clean, tepid water. In most cases, the eye should be checked by a doctor right after you've washed the damaging liquids out.

‡ CONJUNCTIVITIS (PINK EYE)

Once a day, make a poultice of grated apple or grated raw red potato and place it on your closed eye. Let it stay on for ½ hour. Within 2 days, 3 at the most, the condition should completely clear up.

Prepare camomile tea. When it cools, use it as an eyewash twice a day until the conjunctivitis is gone.

NOTE: Conjunctivitis can be a severe and contagious infection at which a health professional should have a look-see.

‡ INFLAMMATIONS AND IRRITATIONS

Peel and slice an overripe apple. Put the pieces of pulp on your closed eyes, holding the pieces in place with a bandage or strip of cloth. Leave it on at least ½ hour to help alleviate irritation and inflammation.

A poultice of either grated raw Irish potato, fresh mashed papaya pulp or mashed cooked beets is soothing and promotes healing. Leave the poultice on for 15 minutes twice a day.

Reuse used tea bags. Make sure they're moist and cool enough to apply to the closed eyelids for 15 minutes. This remedy is a favorite for models who wake up puffy-eyed.

‡ BLACK EYES

We met a friend who had a shiner. We asked, "Did someone give you a black eye?" He answered, "No. I had to fight for it." Had our friend immediately placed a cool wet cloth on the eye and left it there for 20 minutes, he might have greatly minimized the discoloration.

Apply cold, raw beefsteak to the bruised eye, just like in the movies. Actually, there is some controversy over this remedy, but we have testimonies that say it works.

Make a poultice by mixing 2 tablespoonsful of salt with 2 tablespoonsful of lard. Spread the mixture on a cloth and place it over the bruised eye. This poultice may help eliminate the bruised cells around the eye by stimulating the circulation.

‡ NIGHT BLINDNESS

You know the old joke about carrots being good for your eyes? It's true. Well, you've never seen a rabbit wearing glasses. Eat 2 or 3 carrots a day (raw or cooked) and/or drink a glass of fresh carrot juice. It's excellent for alleviating night blindness.

Eat blueberries when they're in season. They can help restore night vision.

Eat watercress in salads and/or drink watercress tea.

‡ EYESTRAIN

Pinch the ends of your index and middle (second and third) fingers of each hand. Thirty seconds on each finger. If your eyestrain isn't relieved after 2 minutes, do another round of pinching.

Sunflower seeds contain vitamins, iron and calcium that may be extremely beneficial for eyes. Everyday eat about ½ cup of unprocessed (unsalted) shelled seeds. (See "Preparation Guide" for roasting instructions.)

‡ CATARACTS

There are revolutionary new methods of removing cataracts, where the patient walks in and out of the doctor's office within a few hours. While you're checking into today's modern techniques, you might want to try one or more of the following, to give you some relief until the cataract is professionally removed:

Take 15 mg of vitamin B-2 daily. Also, eat foods high in vitamin B-2: broccoli, salmon, beans, wheat germ, turnip tops and beets.

Before bedtime, fill an eyedropper with the fresh juice of a coconut and drop in a few drops so that the juice overflows, really washing the eye with the coconut milk. Follow that up with a warm washcloth on the eye for 15 minutes. (See "Preparation Guide" for instructions on milking a coconut.)

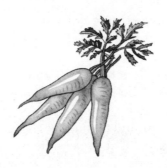

For 5 minutes each day, massage the base of the index and middle (second and third) fingers, as well as the webs between those fingers. The right hand helps the right eye and the left hand helps the left eye.

‡ EYE STRENGTHENERS

Apply cold water on a washcloth to the eyelids, eyebrows and temples morning, noon and night, 5 to 10 minutes each time.

Eat about ½ cup of unprocessed (unsalted) sunflower seeds every day. (See "Preparation Guide" for instructions on roasting the shelled seeds.)

Put a handful of rose petals (the petals are more potent as the flower fades) into a pot and cover with water. Put it over a medium flame. When the water boils, take the pot off the flame and let it cool. Then strain the water into a bottle and close it tight. When your eyes feel tired, weak and red, treat them with the rose petal water. Pour the liquid on a washcloth or cotton pads and keep them on your closed eyes for 15 to 30 minutes. Your outlook might then be a lot rosier.

This is an interesting way to end the day. Prepare a candle, a straight-back chair and a 5-minute timer. Light the candle and place it 1½ feet from you once you're seated in the chair with your feet uncrossed, flat on the floor. The lit candle should be level with the top of your head. Set the timer for 5 minutes. Then, using your index fingers, hold your eyelids open while you stare at the candle without blinking.

There will be tears. Do not wipe them away. Tough out the 5 minutes every other night for 2 weeks. Discontinue the exercise for 2 weeks. Then start again, every other night for 2 weeks. Once your vision is sufficiently strengthened, blow out the candle for good.

‡ EYEWASH FOR BRIGHT, CLEAR EYES

Place a handful of scrubbed carrot tops in a jar of hot water. Let it stand. When it's cool, use the carrot water as an eyewash. Drink the remaining liquid. It should help your eyes and also help strengthen your kidneys and bladder.

Mix 1 drop of lemon juice in 1 ounce of warm water and use it as an eyewash. It's particularly effective when your eyes have been exposed to dust, cigarette smoke, harsh lights and chemical compounds in the air.

‡ SUNBURNED EYES

See "Burns."

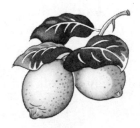

‡Feet

"Oh, my aching feet!" is a common cry heard round the world.

Our feet carry a lot of weight and are probably the most abused and neglected part of our anatomy. At some time or other, we're all guilty of the Cinderella Stepsister syndrome—pushing our feet into ill-fitting shoes.

We put our poor, tired tootsies under all kinds of stress and strain. They get cold, they get frostbitten, they get wet, they burn, they blister, they itch, they sweat, as we walk, jog, run, dance, climb, skate, ski, hop, skip and jump. Then we wonder why our feet are "just killing us!" Well, we killed them first.

Let's get to the bottom of our troubles with some remedies for the feet.

‡ CORNS

The difference between an oak tree and a tight shoe is that one makes acorns, the other makes corns ache. Now, what to do for those aching corns:

Rub castor oil on the corn twice a day and it will gradually peel off, leaving soft, smooth skin.

Every night, put 1 piece of fresh lemon peel on the corn (the inside of the peel on the outside of the corn). Put a Band-Aid around it to keep it in place. In a few days, the corn should be gone.

Make a poultice of 1 crumbled piece of bread soaked in ¼ cup of vinegar. Let it stand for ½ hour, then apply it to the corn and tape it in place overnight. By morning, the corn should peel off. If it's a particularly stubborn corn, you may have to reapply the bread/vinegar poultice a few nights in a row.

Every day, wrap a strip of fresh pineapple peel around the corn (the inside of the peel taped directly on the corn). Within a week, the corn should disappear, thanks to the enzymes and acid content of the fresh pineapple.

Hell hath no fury like a woman's corn! Here are a couple of more remedies:

Don't throw away used tea bags. Tape a moist one on the corn for ½ hour a day and the corn should be gone in a week or two.

To ease the pain of a corn, soak the feet in oatmeal water. Bring 5 quarts (20 cups) of water to a boil and add 5 ounces (1⅔ cups) of oatmeal. Keep boiling until the water boils down to about 4 quarts. Then pour off the clear water through a strainer, into a large enough basin for your feet. Soak your feet for at least 20 minutes.

‡Athlete's Foot

The fungus that causes athlete's foot dies in natural sunlight. So, if you can spend the next 2 weeks barefoot in the Bahamas...If that's a bit impractical, then for 1 hour a day, expose your feet to sunlight and that might eliminate a mild case of athlete's foot.

In between sunbaths, keep the feet well-aired by wearing loose-fitting socks. At night, apply alcohol (Ow! it stings for a couple of seconds), then wait till your feet are very dry and sprinkle on talcum powder (the unscented kind is preferable).

Apply 1 clove of crushed garlic to the affected area. Leave it on for ½ hour, then wash with water. If you do this once a day, within a week, you'll be smelling like a salami, but you may not have athlete's foot.

CAUTION: When you first apply the garlic, there will be a sensation of warmth for a few minutes. If after a few minutes, that warm feeling intensifies and the garlic is burning the skin, wash the area with cool water. Next day, dilute garlic juice with water and try again.

Every evening, apply cotton or cheesecloth that has been saturated with honey to the infected area. Tape it in place. To avoid a gooey mess (a possibility even with the tape in place), wear socks to bed. In the morning, wash with water, dry thoroughly and sprinkle on (preferably unscented) talcum powder. In a week's time, you may have every bear in the neighborhood at your feet, but they probably won't be athlete's foot feet.

To avoid reinfecting yourself with athlete's foot, soak your socks and hose in vinegar. Also wipe out your shoes with vinegar.

‡ ACHING FEET

During a busy day when your "dogs are barking" and you feel like you're going to have to call it quits, cayenne pepper to the rescue! Sprinkle some cayenne into your socks, or rub it directly on the soles of your aching feet. Now get going or you'll be late for your next appointment!

After a long day, when your nerves are on edge, your feet hurt, you're tired—too tired to go to sleep —soak your feet in hot water for 10 to 15 minutes. Then (this is the important part) massage your feet with lemon juice. After you've done a thorough job of massaging, rinse your feet with cool water. As always, dry your feet completely, then take 5 deep breaths. You and your painless feet should be ready and able to settle down for a good night's sleep.

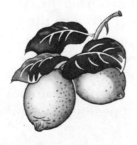

‡ BURNING FEET

Wrap tomato slices on the soles of the feet and keep the feet elevated for ½ hour.

Boil 4 scrubbed potatoes in 6 pints of water until the potatoes are soft. Then remove them from the water. When the water cools a bit, soak the feet in it for 15 minutes. Dry the feet thoroughly. If you're going right to bed, massage the feet with a small amount of sesame or almond oil. You might want to put on loose-fitting socks to avoid messing up the sheets.

Bavarian mountain climbers, after soaking their feet in potato water, sprinkle hot, roasted salt on a cloth and wrap it around their feet. It not only soothes burning and tired feet, but relieves itchy ones as well.

‡ COLD FEET

Stand on your toes for a couple of minutes, then quickly come back down on your heels. Repeat toes/heels several times until your blood tingles through your feet and warms them up.

Before going to bed, walk in cold water in the bathtub for 2 minutes. Then briskly rub the feet dry with a coarse towel. To give the feet a warm glow, hold each end of the towel and run it back and forth through the hollow of the feet.

If the thought of putting already cold feet into cold water is not appealing to you, then add 1 cup of table salt to a bathtub filled, ankle-high, with hot water and soak the feet for 15 minutes. Dry the feet and massage them with damp salt. This will remove dead skin and stimulate circulation. After you've rubbed each foot for 3 to 5 minutes, rinse them both in lukewarm water and dry them thoroughly.

Sprinkle cayenne pepper into your socks before putting them on. They will, of course, turn red—your socks and your feet—the latter will also feel warm. If you're at a restaurant and the food is too bland, take off a sock and season to taste.

‡ **PIGEON-TOED**

If you are slightly pigeon-toed and an orthopedist hasn't helped you, as a last resort, buy a pair of shoes one size larger than you usually take. Wear them to bed every night with the right shoe on the left foot and the left shoe on the right foot. It may not help correct your feet, but it might make you a more interesting person.

‡Female Problems

We've come a long way, baby!

Today, we talk openly about menstruation, pregnancy and menopause, not as sicknesses, but as natural stages of life. We also recognize and deal with premenstrual tension, menstrual pain and menopausal irregularities.

And, we are finally learning to question the male-dominated medical profession after hearing countless stories about hysterectomies, radical mastectomies and other surgery that's sometimes performed whether a woman needs it or not.

Remember, knowledge is power. Television talk shows, book stores and local libraries are filled with women's health information. Take advantage of these sources so that you can intelligently and happily take responsibility for your own body, your choices for professional medical care and for good health.

Meanwhile, here are some home remedies whispered down from generation to generation.

‡ BRINGING ON MENSTRUATION

NOTE: NONE OF THESE REMEDIES WILL WORK IF YOU ARE PREGNANT.

To help bring on and regulate menstruation, eat and drink fresh beets and beet juice. Have about 3 cups of beets and juice each day past your due-date until the flow begins.

A foot bath in hot water has been said to bring on a delayed menstrual period.

Add 1 tablespoonful of basil to a cup of boiling water. Let it steep for 5 minutes. Strain and drink.

In a circular motion, massage below the outer and inner ankle of each foot, as well as the outer and inner wrist of each hand. If there is tenderness when you rub those areas, you're in the right place. Keep massaging until the tenderness is gone. Chances are your problem will also soon be gone. Within a day or two, your period should start.

Ginger tea can stimulate the onset of menstruation. Put 2 or 3 nickel-size pieces of fresh ginger in a cup of hot, not boiling, water and let it steep for 10 minutes. Drink 3 or 4 cups of the tea throughout the day. It also helps ease menstrual cramps.

‡ EXCESSIVE MENSTRUAL FLOW

NOTE: Hemorrhaging requires immediate medical attention! If you are not sure about the difference between hemorrhaging and excessive menstrual flow, do not take a chance—if you are bleeding profusely, get medical attention quickly. If your menstrual flow is excessive, the following remedies have been said to help. We also suggest you have a checkup.

Mix the juice of ½ lemon into a cup of warm water. Drink it down slowly an hour before breakfast and an hour before dinner.

Throughout the day, sip cinnamon tea made with a piece of cinnamon stick steeped in hot water. Or use 4 drops of cinnamon bark tincture in a cup of warm water.

When bleeding excessively, stay away from alcoholic beverages and hot, spicy foods, except for cayenne pepper. (See next remedy.)

Add ⅛ of a teaspoonful of cayenne pepper to a cup of warm water or your favorite herbal tea and drink it. Cayenne pepper is a powerful bleeding regulator.

To help control profuse menstrual flow, it's time for thyme tea. Steep 2 tablespoonsful of thyme in 2 cups of hot water. Let it stand for 10 minutes. Strain and drink 1 cup. Add an ice cube to the other cup of tea, then soak a washcloth in it and use it as a cold compress on the pelvic area.

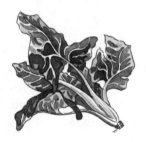

‡ PREMENSTRUAL TENSION AND PERIOD PAINS

Camomile tea is a superb tension reliever and nerve relaxer. As soon as menstrual cramps start, prepare camomile tea and sip it throughout the day.

Premenstrual tension as well as menstrual cramps may be relieved by increasing calcium intake. Menopausal symptoms may also be prevented by adding calcium to the diet. On a daily basis, it is a good idea to eat at least one portion of a minimum of one of these calcium-rich foods: beans (lentil, aduki, chickpeas, etc.) and leafy green vegetables (watercress, kale, parsley, endive, mustard greens). While dairy products have calcium, we feel better when we concentrate on beans and leafy greens for our calcium supply.

Peppermint tea is soothing. It also helps digestion and rids you of that bloated feeling. Drink a cup of peppermint tea after (not during) your meal.

For premenstrual relief for everything from the blues to breast tenderness, take 2 capsules of garlic daily and/or mix 1 teaspoonful of garlic powder in a cup of warm water. Add honey to taste and drink it at the first sign of premenstrual tension.

‡ MENOPAUSE

A Viennese gynecologist has reported positive results among his female patients treated with bee pollen. Bee pollen contains a combination of male and female hormones. It has been known to help some women do away with or minimize the hot flashes.

DOSE: 3 bee pollen pills (500 mg) a day. If, after a few weeks, you're feeling a lot less menopausal, continue taking the pollen. If you're not less nervous and if the hot flashes have not subsided, then pollen isn't working for you.

If you have excessive menstrual flow during menopause, mix 1 ounce of grated nutmeg in 1 pint of Jamaican rum.

DOSE: Take 1 teaspoonful 3 times a day for the duration of your period.

Eat a cucumber every day. Cukes are said to contain beneficial hormones.

‡ CYSTITIS

Pour a small box of baking soda into a bath of warm water and soak in it for at least a half hour, then rinse under the shower.

Even some physicians now prescribe cranberry juice for cystitis. You can get juice that's sugarless with no added preservatives at most supermarkets, or you can buy cranberry concentrate (which needs to be diluted) at health food stores.

DOSE: One 8-ounce glass in the morning, before breakfast, and 1 glass in the late afternoon. Make sure it's at room temperature, not chilled.

Take 2 garlic capsules a day and, if you don't mind smelling like a salami, drink garlic tea throughout the day. Mash a couple of garlic cloves into hot water and let them steep for 5 minutes. You can also make garlic tea with 1 teaspoonful of garlic powder in hot water.

NOTE: Persistent cystitis may require antibiotics prescribed by a doctor. If that is the case, be sure to eat yogurt with live or active cultures, during and after taking the antibiotics. (See "Yogurt" in the "Home-remedy Starter Kit" chapter.)

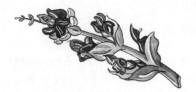

‡ FEMALE PROBLEMS IN GENERAL

Gently but firmly, massage the back of the leg, around the ankle. Massaging that area can relax tension, stimulate circulation and soothe the female organs.

‡ VAGINITIS (INFECTIONS)

Wear cotton panties to absorb moisture, since moisture encourages the growth of organisms. For that reason, stay away from moisture-inducing garments like pantyhose and girdles.

Take showers instead of baths. Baths can add to your problems when the vaginal area is exposed to bathwater impurities.

Do not use any chemical products such as feminine hygiene sprays. Also, avoid tampons and colored toilet tissue.

Do not launder panties along with socks, stockings or other undergarments. Wash panties separately with a mild soap or detergent and rinse them very thoroughly.

Place a poultice of cottage cheese, or farmer cheese, or yogurt with active cultures on a sanitary napkin and wear it. Change the poultice every 3 to 5 hours. Hopefully, the itching will stop rather quickly and the infection will be gone within a week or two.

‡ FRIGIDITY

Frigidity often stems from a lack of communication between a woman and her man. Sex counseling may be necessary. For more information, contact the American Association of Sex Educators, Counselors and Therapists, in Washington, DC.

As for the "Not tonight, honey" syndrome, eating a piece of halvah may awaken sexual desires. This Middle Eastern treat is made of sesame seeds and honey. The sesame seeds are high in magnesium and potassium. Honey has aspartic acid. All 3 substances have been said to help women overcome lack of lust.

Licorice has female hormones in it. In France it might not be uncommon to see women drink licorice water, believing it may improve their love life. Powdered licorice is available at health food stores. Drink 1 teaspoonful in a cup of water and get out the black lingerie.

‡ PREGNANCY: DURING AND AFTER

Morning Sickness

If you are troubled by morning sickness, check with your obstetrician about taking 50 mg of vitamin B-6 and 50 mg of vitamin B-1, daily. Since garlic greatly increases the body's absorption of B-1, make an effort to eat it raw in salads and to cook with it.

Constipation During Pregnancy

Keep a chair, stool or carton in the bathroom so that you can rest your feet on it when you're on the toilet seat. Once your feet are on the same level as the seat, lean back and relax. To avoid hemorrhoids and varicose veins, do not strain and do not hold your breath and squeeze.

Increase Mother's Milk After Pregnancy
Bring to a boil 1 teaspoonful of caraway seeds in 8 ounces of water. Then, simmer for 5 minutes. Let it cool and drink. Several cups of caraway seed tea a day may increase mother's milk supply.

‡Frostbite

The extent of frostbite varies greatly, depending on the length of time a person has been exposed to the cold; the intensity of the cold, humidity, winds; the kinds and amount of clothing worn; a person's natural resistance to cold, as well as a person's general health.

One big problem with frostbite is that it's hard to know you have it until it's on its way to being serious.

At some ski resorts, the ski patrol does occasional nose and cheek checks of skiers. Thanks to those checks, lots of mild frostbite victims are sent indoors to defrost.

Seriously frostbitten victims should be placed under doctor's care and/or hospitalized immediately.

Be sure the frostbite sufferer is in a warm room while waiting for medical help. If he or she is conscious, give him or her a warm drink. NO ALCOHOLIC BEVERAGES! They can worsen the condition. The frozen body parts must be warmed slowly. Be careful when touching the skin not to break the frostbite blisters. Cover the frostbitten areas with a blanket or warm (not hot) water. If it's warm, running water, make sure it runs gently over the skin.

For mild cases of frostbite, all of the above apply; in addition, the following remedies are worth a try.

Steep a teaspoonful of sage in a cup of hot water for 5 minutes and drink it. Sage tea will help improve circulation.

When we were kids, we saw a cartoon of a male Eskimo urinating ice cubes. We didn't see the humor in it. We took it seriously. We have since learned that no matter how cold we are, our urine stays fairly warm. If you're indoors and without warm water, apply your own urine to your frostbitten areas. It should help you thaw out.

Pour witch hazel over the frostbitten areas.

Warm some olive oil and gently dab it on the frostbitten skin or paint it on with a kitchen pastry brush.

Boil and mash potatoes. Add salt and apply the mixture to the frostbitten areas. If you're hungry, eat the potatoes and apply the warm water in which the potatoes were boiled to the frostbitten areas.

‡Hair

According to a French proverb, "A fool's hair never turns white." The Russians say, "There was never a saint with red hair." An American Negro proverb offers this warning: "Don't comb your hair at night; it will make you forgetful." "Pull out a gray hair," according to the German Pennsylvanians, "and seven will come to its funeral."

Hair is a secondary sex characteristic and seems to, appropriately, play a part in sexual attractiveness.

The biggest hair worries: too much or too little. Too much hair, especially in the wrong places, can be permanently removed by electrolysis. It's expensive and painful, but worth every penny and pain in exchange for a better self-image.

Too little hair, especially in men, is usually hereditary baldness (alopecia). Most of our research sources concur that aside from cosmetic surgery (implants and transplants), nothing can be done to restore lost hair.

But wait! We have heard of some unconventional remedies that claim to stop the loss of hair as well as restore the hair already lost. What do you have to lose that you aren't already losing?

‡ STOPPING LOSS AND PROMOTING GROWTH

An hour before bedtime, slice open a clove of garlic and rub it on the hairless area. An hour later, massage the scalp with olive oil, put on a slumber cap and go to bed. Next morning, shampoo. Repeat the procedure night and morning for a few weeks and, hopefully, hair will have stopped falling out and there will be a regrowth showing.

Three times a day, 5 minutes each time, buff your fingernails with your fingernails. Huh? In other words, rub the fingernails of your right hand across the fingernails of your left hand. Not only is it supposed to stop hair loss, it's also supposed to encourage hair growth and prevent hair from graying.

Prepare your own hair-growing elixir by combining ¼ cup of onion juice with 1 tablespoonful of honey. Massage the scalp with the mixture every day. We heard about a man who had a bottle of this hair tonic. One day, he took the cork out of the bottle with his teeth. Next day, he had a mustache that needed to be trimmed.

DO NOT DO THIS EXERCISE IF YOU HAVE HIGH OR LOW BLOOD PRESSURE! Stand on your head. If you can't, then get down on all fours, with your hands about 2 feet from your knees. Then carefully lift your rear end in the air so that your legs are straight and your head is between your outstretched arms. Stay in that position for a minute each day, and after a week, gradually work your way up to 5 minutes each day. The theory behind this is that you will bring oxygen to the hair bulbs, which will rejuvenate the scalp and encourage hair to grow.

‡ DRY HAIR

Shampoo and towel-dry your hair. Then, evenly distribute 1 tablespoonful of mayonnaise throughout your hair. (Use more if your hair is long.) After the mayonnaise has been on an hour, wash hair with a mild shampoo and rinse. The theory is that the flow of oil from the sebaceous glands is encouraged as the natural fatty acids of the mayonnaise help nourish the hair.

‡ FRIZZY DRY HAIR

After shampooing, rinse with 1 tablespoonful of wheat germ oil, followed by a mixture of ½ cup of apple cider vinegar and 2 cups of water. It will tame the frizzies.

‡ DULL, LIFELESS HAIR

After shampooing, rinse with a combination of 1 cup of apple cider vinegar and 2 cups of water. Your hair will come alive and shine. This treatment is especially effective on lifeless permed hair.

‡ THIN, BODILESS HAIR

Add 2 egg whites and the juice of ½ lemon to your shampoo. This will give your hair more body and volume.

‡ DANDRUFF

Wash your hair with a combination of 1 cup of beet juice and 2 cups of water, plus 1 teaspoonful of salt. This is an Arabian remedy. Remember, Arabs have dark hair. Since beets contain a dye, this is not recommended for light-haired people who want to stay that way. To be safe, do a test on a patch of hair.

Squeeze the juice of 1 large lemon and apply half of it to your hair. Mix the other half with 2 cups of water. Wash your hair with a mild shampoo, then rinse with water. Rinse again with the lemon and water mixture. Repeat every other day until dandruff disappears.

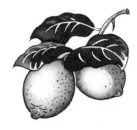

‡Headaches

Take a holistic approach to yourself and your headache. Step back and look at the past 24 hours of your life. Have you eaten sensibly? Did you get a decent night's sleep? Have you moved your bowels since awakening this morning? Are there deadlines you need to meet? Do you have added pressures at home or at work? Is there something you're dreading?

Now that you probably realize the reason for your headache, what should you take for it? Don't refuse any offer.

Since studies show that more than 90% of headaches are brought on by nervous tension, most of our remedies are for the common tension headache and a few for the more serious migraines.

In the case of regularly recurring headaches, they can be caused by eyestrain, an allergy, or something more serious. We suggest you seek professional medical attention.

Headaches are a headache! Use your instincts, common sense and patience to find what works best for you and your headache.

‡ HEADACHES IN GENERAL

When our grandmother had a headache, she would dip a large white handkerchief in vinegar, wring it out and tie it tightly around her forehead until the headache disappeared.

A variation of soaking a handkerchief in vinegar is to soak a brown paper bag in vinegar. Shake off the excess liquid and place it on your forehead. Tie it in place for at least ½ hour.

Peel the rind off a lemon. Make the pieces as wide as possible. Rub the rind (the inside of the skin should touch your skin) on your forehead and temples. Then place the rind on the forehead and temples, securing them with a scarf or bandage. Keep it there until the headache goes away.

Let ice-cold water accumulate, ankle-high, in the bathtub. Dress warmly except for your bare feet. Take a leisurely stroll in the tub—from 1 to 5 minutes—as long as it takes for your feet to start feeling warm in the ice-cold water. When that happens, get out of the tub and go directly to bed. Cover up, relax and within no time, your headache should be a pain of the past.

Press your thumb against the roof of your mouth for 4 to 5 minutes. Every so often, move your thumb to another section of the roof of your mouth. The nerve pressure in your head should be greatly relieved. However, it's highly impractical during a speaking engagement.

Mix a cup of water with a cup of apple cider vinegar and bring it to a slow boil in a medium-size pot. When the fumes begin to rise, reduce the flame as low as it will get. Put a towel over your head, bend over the pot and inhale exhale deeply through your nose about 80 times or for about 10 minutes. Make sure you hold the towel so that it doesn't catch fire, but catches the vapor for you to inhale.

If strawberries are in season, eat a few. They contain organic salicylates, which are like the active ingredients in aspirin.

Vigorously rub the second joint of each thumb, 2 minutes on the right hand, 2 minutes on the left hand, until you've done it five times each, or for 10 minutes. Use hand lotion on the thumbs to eliminate friction.

A very old American remedy is a teaspoonful of honey mixed with ½ teaspoonful of garlic juice.

During my est training, I was told that whatever you fully experience, disappears. This est process can help you experience away your headache. Ask yourself the following questions and answer them honestly:

- Do you *really* want to get rid of the headache? (Don't laugh. A lot of people want to hang on to their headaches. It's a great excuse and cop-out from all kinds of things.)
- What kind of headache is it? Be specific. Is it a pounding over one eye? Does it throb each time you bend down? Do you have a dull ache at the base of your neck? Now, either learn the next questions by heart or have someone read them to you. ("Why?" you wonder.) Close your eyes. ("Aha!" That's why.)
- What size is your headache? Describe the exact dimensions of it. Start with the length from the front of your face to the back of your head, the width from ear to ear and the thickness of it.

- What color is your headache?
- How much water will it hold? (This is done in your mind through visualization.) Fill a cup with the amount of water needed to fill the area of the headache. Then, pour the water from the cup into the space of your headache. When you've completed that, open your eyes. You should have experienced away your headache. The first time I used this process, my results were quite dramatic. If I hadn't experienced it myself, I'd probably think it's as crazy as you're probably thinking I am right now.

‡ SINUS HEADACHES

Sniff a little horseradish juice—the stronger the horseradish, the better. Remember to do it slowly.

Prepare poultices of either raw grated onion or horseradish. Apply the poultices to the nape of the neck and the soles of the feet. Leave them on for an hour.

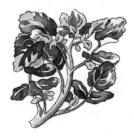

‡ MIGRAINES

Dip a few cabbage leaves in boiling hot water to make them soft. As soon as they're cool enough, place 1 or 2 thicknesses on your forehead and on the back of your neck. Secure them in place with a scarf or bandage. Then relax as the cabbage draws out the pain.

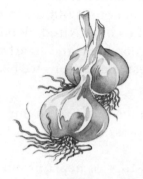

Boil 2 Spanish onions. Eat 1 and mash the other for a poultice. Then place it on your head.

Apply pressure to the palm of one hand with the thumb of the other hand. Then, reverse the order. If you feel a tenderness in either palm, concentrate the massage on that area. Keep up the firm pressure and massage for 10 minutes—5 minutes on each hand.

We heard about a woman who would take a tablespoonful of honey the second she felt a migraine coming on. If the headache wasn't gone within a half-hour, she'd take another tablespoonful of honey with 3 glasses of water and that would do it.

NOTE: Chronic migraine sufferers should seek medical attention.

‡Heart

The heart is a four-chambered hollow muscle and double-acting pump located in the chest between the lungs. This hard-working, fist-size muscle pumps blood through the blood vessels in all parts of the body at the rate of about 4,000 gallons a day. (No wonder so many of us have 'tired blood.')

The heart is so complex and heart trouble is so serious that the best suggestions we can offer are:

- If you feel as though you're having a heart attack, call for professional medical help IMMEDIATELY!
- If you have a history of heart problems, follow an eating plan that will promote a healthy heart. Look into the American Heart Association Diet (it's in book form); the macrobiotic way of eating (for information call the Kushi Foundation in Brookline, Massachusetts); and a learn-by-doing program of living foods and wheatgrass therapy at the Hippocrates Health Institute (Boston, Massachusetts).
- To help others, take a cardiac pulmonary resuscitation (CPR) course through your local Red Cross chapter.

While doing research, we found some things that may help strengthen the heart. We'd like to share them with you, with the understanding that these *do not* take the place of professional medical attention.

Eat lots of alfalfa sprouts every day—in soups, on sandwiches and in salads. Grow your own sprouts. (See "Preparation Guide" for growing instructions.) Alfalfa is wonderful for helping to dissolve cholesterol deposits.

For a healthier heart, eat wheat germ every day. You might want to supplement the wheat germ with vitamin E (400 I.U.). It's said to help reduce hardening of the arteries.

If you have palpitations occasionally, as most of us do, drink peppermint tea. Have a mugful a day. It seems to have a calming effect on people, especially since it is an herb tea that does not have caffeine.

Take 2 capsules of garlic a day to protect and strengthen the heart and help thin the blood. Also, use garlic in cooking and raw in salads.

According to wine therapists, a little champagne or dry light wine sipped daily helps strengthen the heart. (Please remember, EVERYTHING IN MODERATION!) The champagne's tartrate of potassium content supposedly has a positive effect on one's cardiac rhythm.

We've been told that massaging the pads at the base of the last 2 fingers of the left hand, or massaging the left foot under the third, fourth and fifth toes, can relieve heart pain within seconds.

If someone wants to give you an edible treat, instead of candy suggest red roses. They're said to help strengthen the heart as well as other organs of the body, not to mention what they do for a relationship. Remove the bitter white part on the bottom of the petals and eat the rest of the petals raw, or make rose petal tea to drink. There are tribes in India who live on roses alone. They don't have their groceries delivered. They send flowers by wire.

Eat onions once a day. According to Russian scientists, onions are good for all kinds of heart problems.

Every morning, before breakfast, drink the juice of half a lemon in a cup of warm water. It's reputed to be helpful for all kinds of body functions from proper fluid action in the blood to regularity in the bathroom.

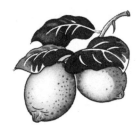

‡Hemorrhoids (Piles)

Hemorrhoids, or piles, are varicose veins in or around the rectum. It is truly a pain in the anus.

Two out of every three adults have had, currently have or will have hemorrhoids. Chances are, if you're reading this page, you are one of the two out of the three.

Along with treating your condition with natural, non-chemical remedies, here are ways of speeding up the healing process:

• Keep the bowels as clear as possible. Drink lots of fruit juices and vegetable juices. Stay away from hard-to-digest, overly-processed foods: white flour, sugar, alcoholic beverages, etc.
• Do not strain or hold your breath while having a bowel movement. Make an effort to breathe evenly.
• Take a brisk walk as often as you can, especially after meals.

Heed the suggestions above as well as the ones on the following pages, and hopefully, in a few days, you'll have this problem behind you.

Take 100 mg of rutin 3 times a day. This has helped hemorrhoid sufferers when all else has failed.

Apply liquid lecithin directly on the hemorrhoids, once a day, until they completely disappear.

Eat a large boiled leek every day as an afternoon snack or with dinner. Eat 3 raw unprocessed almonds every day. Chew each one about 50 times.

Insert a peeled clove of garlic in the rectum right after a bowel movement. Keep it in as long as possible. Then, before bedtime, insert another peeled clove, as high as you can push it with your finger. In order to keep it in overnight, you might have to put on a T-bandage. Garlic should help reduce the swelling quite quickly. Repeat the procedure daily until you're hemorrhoid-free.

Put a cottage cheese poultice on the hemorrhoid area to help relieve pain. Change the poultice 3 times a day.

Put ¼ cup of cranberries in a blender so that they're finely chopped. Place 1 tablespoonful in a piece of cheesecloth and insert it in the rectum. An hour later, remove the cheesecloth insert and replace it with another tablespoonful of chopped cranberries in cheesecloth for another hour. This is a great pain reliever. By the end of 2 hours, you should feel much better.

Cut a peeled, raw potato in the shape of a suppository (like a bullet) and insert it in the rectum. This folk remedy has had dramatic positive results.

Add ¼ cup of witch hazel to a basin of warm water. Sit in it for at least 15 minutes at a time, at least 2 times a day. Complete cures have been reported within 3 days.

Psychic healer, Edgar Cayce, recommended this exercise to a hemorrhoid sufferer:

1. Stand with feet about 6 inches apart. Hands at sides.
2. Raise your hands up to the ceiling.
3. Bend forward and bring your hands as close to the floor as you can.
4. Go back to the first position.

Repeat the entire procedure 3 dozen times. It should take just a few minutes to do. Do it an hour after breakfast and an hour after dinner, every day until the hemorrhoids are history.

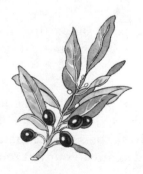

‡Hiccups

A hiccup is a spastic contraction of the diaphragm —the large circular muscle that separates the chest from the abdomen.

Hiccups are a great conversation starter. If you're in a room with 30 people, ask each one of them how they get rid of the hiccups and you will probably get 30 different remedies.

According to the *Guinness Book of World Records*, the longest recorded attack of hiccups is that afflicting Charles Osborne of Iowa. He was born in 1894 and got the hiccups in 1922, when he was 28. He still has them as of the printing of the 1983 revised *Guinness Book* edition. The hiccups started while Mr. Osborne was slaughtering a hog. He has hiccupped about 420 million times since then.

To prevent a case of the hiccups, do not slaughter a hog. To cure a case of the hiccups, try one or more of the following remedies.

NOTE: there are some medications available to help stop chronic hiccupping.

Drink a glass of pineapple or orange juice.

Make believe your index finger is a mustache. Place it under your nose and press in hard for 30 seconds.

Drink a glass of water that has a tablespoon in it—the bowl of the spoon being the part that's in the water. As you drink, be sure the metal handle of the spoon is pressed against your left temple.

Swallow a teaspoonful of fresh onion juice.

Mix a teaspoonful of apple cider vinegar in a cup of warm water and drink it down.

Drink a glass of water from the far side of the glass. You have to bend far forward to do this without dribbling all over yourself.

Gently inhale a little pepper—enough to make you sneeze a couple of times. Sneezing usually makes the hiccups disappear.

Eat a piece of dry bread (a few days old, if possible). Chew each bite thoroughly. By the time you finish the slice of bread, the hiccups should be gone.

When children between the ages of seven and fourteen have the hiccups, promise to double their allowance if they can hiccup once more after you say "Go!" Chances are there will not be one more hiccup after you say, "Go!" We don't know why, but it works.

Place an ice cube right below the Adam's apple and count to 150.

Take a mouthful of water and keep it in your mouth while you stick the middle fingers of each hand into your ears and press fairly firmly. Count to 100, then swallow the water and unplug your ears.

Pretend you're singing at the Metropolitan Opera House without a microphone and the foremost opera critic is in the last row of the uppermost tier. One aria and the hiccups should disappear. (So might your roommate.)

Take 7 drinks of water without taking a breath in between swallows. While you're drinking the water, turn the glass to the left.

Put a handkerchief over a glass of water and suck the water through it as you would with a straw.

Stick out your tongue as far as possible and keep it out for 3 minutes. Be careful, one big hiccup and—ouch!

The sole of the foot is an acupressure point for curing the hiccups. Massage the center of the sole for as long as it takes for the hiccups to stop.

Mix ½ teaspoonful of sugar in ½ glass of water and drink it slowly.

Place a pencil between your teeth so that it sticks out on both sides of your mouth. Chomp down on it while drinking a glass of water.

If nothing else works, take a hot bath. This has helped cure severe cases of hiccups.

‡Indigestion

Mae West said, "Too much of a good thing is wonderful!" We say, "Too much of a good thing can cause indigestion!"

There are different types of indigestion: mild, severe and persistent. Persistent indigestion may be a food allergy. Get professional medical help to check it out. Severe indigestion may be something a lot more serious than you think. Seek professional help immediately.

CAUTION: NEVER TAKE A LAXATIVE WHEN YOU HAVE SEVERE STOMACH PAIN.

Mild indigestion usually produces one or a combination of the following symptoms: stomach ache, heartburn, nausea and vomiting, or gas.

The first thing a person suffering from a mild case of indigestion usually does is promise never to overindulge again. That takes care of next time. As for now, relief is just a page or two away.

‡ INDIGESTION IN GENERAL

By eating 1 large radish, all the symptoms and discomfort of indigestion may disappear, unless radishes do not agree with you, in which case, move on to the next remedy.

Mix 1 tablespoonful of honey and 2 teaspoonsful of apple cider vinegar into a glass of hot water and drink the mixture.

Put on a yellow slicker, not because it's raining, but because color therapists claim that the color yellow has rays that can help heal all digestive problems. Eat yellow foods like bananas, lemons, pineapple, squash and grapefruit. Lie down on a yellow sheet and get a massage with some yellow oil. What could be bad?

Camomile and/or peppermint teas are very soothing. At the first sign of indigestion, drink a cup of either one.

Eat, drink or take some form of papaya after eating. Fresh papaya (the *yellow* ones are ripe), papaya juice or papaya pills help combat indigestion, thanks to the potent digestive enzyme they contain called papain.

In moderation, drink some white wine *after*, not during, a meal to help overcome indigestion.

Arrowroot is a wonderful stomach settler. Combine 1 tablespoonful of arrowroot with enough water to make a smooth paste. Boil the mixture. Let it cool, then add 1 tablespoonful of lime juice and take it when you have "agita."

Garlic helps stimulate the secretion of digestive enzymes. If you're plagued by indigestion, take 2 garlic pills after lunch and after dinner. Use garlic in salads and in cooking whenever possible, unless garlic *gives* you indigestion.

Scrub an orange and eat some of the peel 5 minutes after a meal.

Boiled or steamed zucchini sprinkled with raw grated almonds is a side dish with your meal that will ensure better digestion.

Alfalfa seed tea is an effective stomach settler. Bring to a boil 1 teaspoonful of alfalfa seed in 1 cup of water. Then let it steep for 5 minutes. Drink it ½ hour after you've eaten.

Cayenne pepper sprinkled sparingly (no more than ¼ teaspoonful) on food or in soup, will aid digestion.

Add basil to food while cooking. It will make the food more digestible and also help prevent constipation. If you really have a taste for basil, add ⅛ to ¼ teaspoonful to a glass of white wine and drink it *after*, not during, the meal.

If you have trouble digesting raw vegetables, at least 3 hours before eating, sprinkle the veggies with fresh lemon juice. Somehow the lemon, as wild as this sounds, partly digests the hard-to-digest parts of the greens.

‡ STOMACH CRAMPS
Steep 1 teaspoonful of fresh or dried parsley in 1 cup of hot water. After 5 minutes, strain and slowly

drink the parsley tea. Remember that parsley tea also acts as a diuretic, so make sure you plan accordingly, because you may have to "eat and run."

Slice 1 medium-size onion and boil it in 1 cup of milk. Drink this concoction warm. It sounds awful and probably is, but it's an old home remedy that may work.

Water has amazing healing power. Get in a hot shower and let the water beat down on your stomach for 10 to 15 minutes. By the time you dry off, you should be feeling a lot better.

American Indians used this one for tum-tum aches: Pour 1 cup of boiling water over 1 teaspoonful of cornmeal. Let it sit for 5 minutes. Add salt to taste and drink slowly.

‡ NAUSEA AND VOMITING

Always keep a bottle of ginger ale in the refrigerator. When you feel nauseated, drink about ½ cup of the soda. One or two burps later, you'll feel fine again.

Drink a cup of camomile tea to calm the stomach and stop vomiting.

A couple of cloves steeped in boiling water for 5 minutes may do the trick, after you've drunk it, of course. If the taste of cloves reminds you too much of the dentist, then steep a piece of cinnamon stick in boiling water, or 1 teaspoonful of powdered ginger. All of them are fine for stopping nausea and vomiting.

Crack an ice cube and suck on the little pieces. It's worth a try when you have nothing else in the house.

This remedy is the pits—the armpits. Peel a large onion and cut it in half. Place each half under each armpit. We've been told it stops vomiting and relieves nausea in no time.

If you're outside, feeling nauseated inside, stop at the nearest luncheonette and ask for a teaspoonful of pure cola syrup with a water chaser.

‡ HEARTBURN

Whatever you do, don't lie down when you have heartburn. Instead, stay on your feet and try one of the following:

Eat ½ dozen blanched almonds. Chew each one at least 30 times.

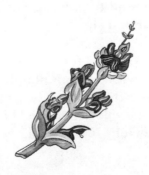

Eat a slice of raw potato.

Or: Grate a raw potato and put it in cheesecloth. Squeeze out the juice in a glass. Add twice the amount of warm water as potato juice and drink it down.

Mix 1 tablespoonful of apple cider vinegar and 1 tablespoonful of honey into a cup of warm water. Stir and drink.

Peel and eat a raw carrot. Chew each biteful 30 times.

If you have heartburn from eating something sweet, squeeze ½ lemon into a cup of warm water. Add ½ teaspoonful of salt and drink it slowly.

‡ GAS/FLATULENCE

A strong cup of peppermint tea will give you relief very quickly, especially if you walk around as you drink it.

A hot water compress placed directly on the stomach can relieve gas pains.

Add 1 teaspoonful of anisette liqueur to a cup of warm water. Stir and sip.

An old home remedy for gas and heartburn is a raw onion sandwich. Some people would rather *have* gas and heartburn than eat a raw onion sandwich, and some people *get* gas and heartburn from a raw onion sandwich. If onions agree with you, it's worth a try.

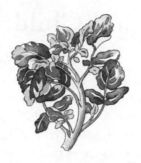

Add ½ teaspoonful of bay leaves to a cup of boiling water. Let it cook, then strain it and drink it down slowly.

Get rid of a gas condition with mustard seeds and lots of water. The first day take 2 seeds; the second day take 4 and so on until you take 12 seeds on the sixth day. Then work it down to 2 seeds on the eleventh day. By then you should be fine. Continue to take 2 seeds a day. Always take the mustard seeds on an empty stomach.

‡ BELCHING
This is a Taoist remedy that dates back to the sixth century B.C. Scrub a tangerine, then peel it and boil the pieces of peel for 5 minutes. Strain, let cool and drink the tangerine tea. The tea should stop you from belching. You can also eat the tangerine peel as a digestive aid.

‡Infants and Children

Every baby-care book tells you to "childproof" your home. Make a crawling tour of each room in your house in order to see things from a child's-eye view. Once you're aware of the danger zones, you can eliminate them by covering wires, nailing down furniture, etc. Do this every 4 to 6 months as the child grows and is able to reach more things.

Still, no matter how childproof a place is, a mishap can happen. We suggest that parents have a first-aid book handy and/or take a first-aid course through the local American Red Cross.

It's also very important to keep a list of the following emergency numbers near every telephone in the house:
• Pediatrician
• Poison Control Center
• Police
• Fire Department
• Hospital
• Pharmacy
• Dentist
• Neighbors (with cars)

In terms of home remedies for common conditions, we caution you that children's systems are much more delicate than ours. So, while lots of the remedies throughout the book can certainly be applied to youngsters, use good common sense in prescribing doses and strengths. In all cases, check with the pediatrician first.

One major caution: NEVER GIVE HONEY TO A CHILD UNDER ONE YEAR OLD! Spores found in honey have been linked to botulism in babies.

Here are some remedies specifically for children's ailments. They should help you as well as your child to get through those tough times.

‡ BEDWETTING

Give the bedwetter a few pieces of cinnamon bark to chew on throughout the day. For some unknown reason, it seems to control bedwetting.

Prepare a cup of corn silk tea by adding 10 to 15 drops of corn silk extract to a cup of boiled water. Stir, let cool and have the bedwetter slowly sip the tea right before bedtime.

If all else fails, try this: At bedtime, tie a towel around the bedwetter's loins, make sure the knot is in front. This urges the child to sleep on his or her back, which seems to lessen bedwetting urges.

NOTE: Chronic bedwetters should be treated by a health professional.

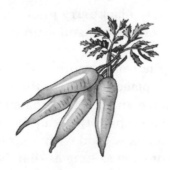

‡ CINDER IN EYE
Irrigate eye with water.

Peel an onion near the child so that tears wash away the cinder.

‡ COUGH
When a child has a bad, hacking cough, spray the pillow with wine vinegar. Both you and the child may sleep better for it.

‡ DIAPER RASH
Let baby's bottom be exposed to the air. If weather permits, the sun (10 to 15 minutes at a time) can do wonders for clearing up diaper rash.

Gently apply honey to the rash. It helps promote healing.

‡ DIARRHEA
Give baby pure blackberry juice.
DOSE: 2 or 3 tablespoonsful 4 times a day.

Carrot soup not only soothes the inflamed small bowel, it also replaces lost body fluids and minerals. Also carrots have an anti-diarrhea substance called pectin. You can prepare the soup by mixing a jar of strained carrots baby food with a jar of water. Feed the child carrot soup as long as diarrhea persists.

Another way of treating diarrhea in infants is to give them barley water throughout the day. (See "Preparation Guide" for the barley water recipe.)

‡ FEVER

To help pull down a child's fever, put sliced, raw potatoes on the soles of the feet and bandage in place. Let the novelty of this remedy provide a few laughs for you and your child. Isn't laughter the best medicine?

‡ HICCUPS

When our friend's six-month-old girl gets the hiccups, Daddy yells at the dog. That makes baby cry. As soon as the baby takes her first deep breath to cry, Daddy quickly cups his hands over her ears and the hiccups stop. (If his dog gets the hiccups, we wonder if he yells at his baby.)

‡ INDIGESTION, COLIC AND GAS

Give your colicky infant mild ginger tea. It's wonderful for digestion and gas problems.

For 15 minutes, boil a cup of water with ⅓ of a bay leaf in the water. Let it cool, then pour it into the baby's bottle and let the baby drink it. This old Sicilian remedy has cured many colicky bambinos.

Mild camomile tea will soothe an upset stomach and calm down colicky kids. That is, if you can calm them down long enough to drink the camomile tea.

If your child seems to have a minor digestion problem, try 2 teaspoonsful of apple juice concentrate in half a glass of water before meals. Make sure the liquid mixture is room temperature, not chilled.

‡ PIGEON-TOES
If your child is slightly pigeon-toed, buy a pair of shoes one size larger than he or she usually takes. Have the child wear them to bed every night with the right shoe on the left foot and the left shoe on the right foot. If there is no improvement within a reasonable amount of time, obviously your child will need more sophisticated treatment.

‡ SPITTING UP
Warm up a little heavy syrup from canned peaches and give it to your baby to stop nausea.

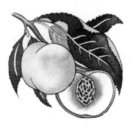

‡ SPLINTERS
To pinpoint the exact location of a splinter, pat some iodine on the area and the sliver of wood will absorb it and turn dark.

Once you've located the splinter, soak the area in vegetable oil for 3 minutes or as long as the child will stay in one place. The oil should allow the splinter to glide right out.

If the child has a sliver of glass, numb the area with an ice cube or some teething lotion before you start the painful squeezing and scraping.

‡ TEETHING

When teething children are being fed, they often cry as though they do not want the food. They may really be hungry but be crying because of the pain caused by a metal spoon. Feed the teething tot with an ivory, wood or bone spoon and make sure the edges are nice and smooth.

Rub the sore little gums with olive oil to help relieve the pain.

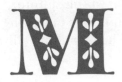

‡Male Problems

It is estimated that one out of every three men over the age of 60 has some kind of prostate problem.

We strongly suggest that if you are suffering with pain, burning, testicular or scrotal swelling, or any other prostate-related symptoms, you have your condition evaluated by a health professional.

As for impotency, most men at some time during their lives experience the dreaded inability to have an erection. That's the bad news. The good news is that it is usually a temporary condition caused by some kind of psychological trauma and emotional tension. While the psyche is being treated with professional help, physical steps can be taken to improve one's sexual energy.

You might want to read through these health hints whether or not anything is bothering you. Chances are you'll find some information you can use to help you maintain your health and sexual potency.

‡ PROSTATE

The prostate contains ten times more zinc than most other organs in the body. Pumpkin seeds have a very high zinc content. That may account for the normalizing effect it is said the seeds have on prostate disorders. It may also be beneficial because of the seeds' iron, phosphorus, vitamins A and B-1, protein, calcium and unsaturated fatty acid content. For whatever reason, pumpkin seeds might have a positive effect on the male genital system.

Eat 3 or 4 palmsful (about ½ cup) of unprocessed (unsalted) shelled pumpkin seeds daily. If you can't get pumpkin seeds, sunflower seeds are second best. Or take zinc tablets—15 mg 2 times a day. For chronic prostate trouble, take 50 mg a day for 6 months, then reduce the dosage to 30 mg a day.

Bee pollen is said to be effective in reducing swelling of the prostate as well as treating other prostate disorders. Pollen contains the hormone testosterone and traces of other male hormones. It seems to give the prostate a boost so that it may heal itself.

DOSE: 5 pollen pills daily—2 in the morning, 2 in the afternoon and 1 in the evening.

Drink 2 to 4 ounces of coconut milk every day to tone up the prostate glands. The milk is pure and uncontaminated and loaded with minerals. It's also a soothing digestive aid. (See "Preparation Guide" for instructions on milking a coconut.)

When the prostate gland is inflamed, apply a watercress poultice to reduce the inflammation.

To relieve prostate pain, in a circular motion, massage the area above the heel and just below the inner ankle of each foot and/or the inside of the wrists, above the palm of each hand. Keep massaging until the pain and soreness disappear.

Prepare parsley tea by steeping a handful of fresh parsley in a cup of hot water for 10 minutes. Drink a few cups of tea throughout the day.

Take hot sitz baths—2 a day. Sit in half a foot of hot water for about 15 minutes. Within a week, inflammation and swelling should be greatly reduced.

Corn silk tea has been a popular folk remedy for prostate problems. Steep a handful of the silky strings that grow around ears of corn, in a cup of hot water for 10 minutes. Drink a few cups throughout the day. If it's not fresh corn season, buy corn silk extract in health food stores, and add 10 to 15 drops in 1 cup of water and drink.

‡ SCROTUM AND TESTICLES

A comfrey poultice applied to the scrotum might reduce swelling and soreness. (See "Poultices" in the "Preparation Guide.")

To relieve testicle pain, massage the outer wrist of each hand and/or the outer ankle of each foot.

‡ MALE PROBLEMS IN GENERAL

To relax tension, stimulate circulation, and generally soothe the male organs, massage the area behind the leg in back of the ankle, about 1 inch or 2 higher than the shoe line of each foot.

‡ IMPOTENCE

According to the teachings of Yogi Bhajan, a man should never have sexual intercourse within 2½ hours after eating a meal, the length of time it takes to digest food.

The sex act is strenuous and requires your mind, your entire nervous system and all your muscles needed for the digestion process. Yogi Bhajan felt that lovemaking right after eating could ruin your stomach and, if done often, could eventually result in premature ejaculation.

While he said that 4 hours between eating and sex is adequate, he thought that for optimal sexual function, a man should have nothing but liquids—juices and soups—24 hours before making love.

Garlic is said to stimulate sexual desire and the production of semen. Eat raw garlic in salads and use it in cooking and take 2 garlic pills a day. Then find a woman who doesn't mind the smell of garlic. By the way, is it a coincidence that the French and Italians have a steady diet of garlic and are said to be vigorous lovers?

Mint is supposed to restore sexual desire. Eat mint leaves and drink mint tea. It's also good for garlic breath.

In Japan, men are advised to firmly squeeze their testicles daily, once for as many years as they are old.

After much research, we've come up with a list of foods some have felt to have aphrodisiacal effects.

At the top of the list is, believe it or not, celery. Eat it every day. Of course, we've all heard about eating oysters. Do! They contain zinc and, like pumpkin seeds, are said to be wonderful for male genitalia. The list continues with peaches, honey, parsley, cayenne pepper, bran cereals and truffles. In fact, Napoleon credited truffles for his ability to sire a son.

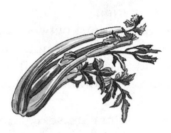

American Indians used ginseng as an aphrodisiac. The Chinese also use ginseng. This herb should be taken sparingly, about ¼ teaspoonful twice a month. It is said to stimulate the endocrine system and be a source of male hormones. Ginseng has also been said to help men who have had a sterility problem.

Contrary to what we've been led to believe about cold showers, they might help stimulate sexual desire. Every day for about 2 months, take a cold shower or cold sitz bath and notice a rejuvenated you.

NOTE: If you have prostate problems, take *hot* sitz baths.

To improve sexual potency, do this yoga exercise before breakfast and before bedtime: Sit on the floor with back straight, head up and feet crossed in front of you. Tighten the muscles in the genital area, including the anus. Count to 20, then relax and count to 20 again. Repeat the procedure 5 times in a row, twice a day.

The English have a commercial preparation called Tonic For Happy Lovers. The recipe consists of combining 1 ounce of licorice root with 2 teaspoonsful of crushed fennel seeds (both of which you should be able to get at a health food store) and 2 cups of water. Bring the mixture to a boil, lower the heat, cover, and simmer slowly for 20 minutes. After it has cooled, strain it and bottle it.

DOSE: 1 to 3 tablespoonsful twice a day.

‡Memory

There seems to be a national epidemic of memory failure. Lately, I hear people of all ages saying things like "I don't remember a thing anymore." "I feel as though I'm losing my mind." "The only thing my memory is good for is to make me wonder what I've forgotten."

There's a vitamin store on the Upper East Side of New York City where the sales clerk offers 2 bottles of Maximum Memory pills at a reduced rate. He also gives you a money-back guarantee if, after finishing the first bottle of pills, your memory hasn't greatly improved. Everyone buys 2 bottles of pills. That's super salesmanship. Think about it. If, after you finish the first bottle, your memory does improve, you will want to keep taking the pills and not return the second bottle. On the other hand, if your memory is still as bad after you've taken the first bottle, chances are you won't remember the salesman's offer, or the place you bought the pills.

It's sort of the same with this chapter. If these memory remedies help, fine. If not, hopefully, you won't remember where you've heard about them.

Choline is used by our brains to make the important chemical acetylcholine, which is required for memory.

At a health food or vitamin store, buy choline chloride or choline hydrochloride, *not* choline bitartrate. (The latter sometimes causes diarrhea.) Taking choline may improve your memory and your ability to learn. You should also notice a keener sense of mental organization.

DOSE: Take 500 mg of choline twice a day. (Set your alarm clock so you won't forget to take it.)

A memory-improving drink: half a glass of carrot juice together with half a glass of milk, daily.

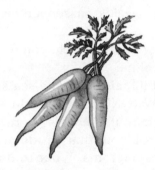

Three prunes a day supposedly improves the memory. It can also help prevent constipation, and since constipation paralyzes the thinking process, take 3 prunes a day.

Daily doses of fresh ginger used in cooking and for tea may heighten the memory.

Add 4 cloves to a cup of sage tea. Sage and cloves have been said to strengthen the memory. Drink a cup every day.

‡Motion Sickness

The story is told about the captain of the ship who announced, "There is no hope. We are all doomed. The ship is sinking and we'll all be dead within an hour." One voice was heard after the announcement. It was the seasick passenger saying, "Thank heavens!"

If you have ever been seasick, you probably anticipated that punchline.

Most people think air, land and sea sickness start in the stomach. WRONG! Guess again. Constant jarring of the semicircular canals in the ears cause inner balance problems that produce those awful motion sickness symptoms. What to do? Go suck a lemon! Really! That's one of the time-tested remedies. There are a few more that might help you get through that miserable feeling.

Before there's a "next time," be sure to read the "And Now May We Prevent" chapter, as well as this one.

Pull out and pinch the skin in the middle of your inner wrist, about an inch from your palm. Keep pulling and pinching alternate wrists until you feel better.

A cup of peppermint or camomile tea may calm down the stomach and alleviate nausea.

Mix ⅛ teaspoonful of cayenne pepper in a cup of warm water or a cup of soup and force yourself to finish it. It won't finish you. It may stop nausea.

At the first sign of motion sickness, take a metal comb or wire brush and run the teeth over the backs of your hands, particularly the area from the thumb to the first finger, including the web of skin in between both fingers. You may have relief in 5 to 10 minutes.

Briskly massage the fourth and fifth fingers of each hand, with particular emphasis on the vicinity of the pinky's knuckle. You may feel relief within 15 minutes; if not, go suck a lemon!

During a bout of motion sickness, suck a lemon or drink some fresh-squeezed lemon juice.

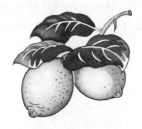

‡Sciatica

Sciatica is a painful condition affecting the sciatic nerve, which is the longest nerve in the body. It extends from the lower spine through the pelvis, thighs, down into the legs and ends at the heels.

We all have some nerve!

The home remedies we describe may not cure the condition, but they may help ease the pain.

The juice from potatoes has been said to help sciatic sufferers. So has celery juice. If you don't have a juicer, your local health food store, one with a juice bar, might be willing to accommodate you. Have them juice a 10-ounce combination of potato and celery juice. Add carrots and/or beets to improve the taste. In addition to the juice, drink a couple of cups of celery tea throughout the day.

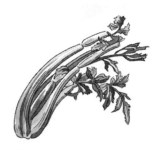

Stimulate the nerve by applying a fresh minced horseradish poultice to the painful area. Keep it on for 1 hour.

According to the *Pakistan Medical Times*, vitamin B-1 and garlic are very beneficial. Eat garlic raw in salads and use it in cooking. Also, take 2 garlic capsules a day, plus 10 mg of vitamin B-1 along with a good vitamin B complex.

A hot water bag may help you make it through the night with less pain and more sleep.

Drink elderberry juice and elderberry tea throughout the day.

Before bedtime, heat olive oil and use it to massage the painful areas.

Eat lots of watercress, parsley and alfalfa sprouts every day.

‡Skin

Skin is the largest organ of the body. The average adult has 17 square feet of skin. Thick or thin skinned, it weighs about 5 pounds.

Five pounds of skin covering 17 square feet of body surface...that's a lot of room for eruptions, cuts, sores, grazes, scrapes, scratches and itches.

Someone named Anonymous once said, "Dermatology is the best specialty. The patient never dies—and never gets well."

Mr. Anonymous said that before reading this chapter.

‡ PIMPLES

Mix the juice of 2 garlic cloves with an equal amount of vinegar and dab it on the pimples every evening. The condition may clear up in a couple of weeks.

Simmer 1 sliced medium onion in ½ cup of honey until the onion is soft. Then mash the mixture into a smooth paste. Make sure it's cool before applying it to blemishes. Leave it on at least 1 hour, then rinse off with warm water. Repeat procedure every evening until "Look Ma, no pimples!"

Eat brown rice regularly. It contains amino acids that are good for skin conditions.

About 4 hours before bedtime, steep 1 cup of mashed strawberries in 2 cups (1 pint) of white vinegar. Let it steep until you're ready for bed. Then strain the pulp and seeds. Massage the remaining liquid on your face and have a good night's sleep. It's not messy as it sounds. The liquid dries on the face before the face touches the pillow. In the morning, wash it off with cool water. This is an excellent cleanser and astringent for blemished skin.

‡ BLACKHEADS
Before going to bed, rub lemon juice over blackheads. Wait until morning to wash off the juice with cool water. Repeat procedure several evenings in a row and you'll see big improvement in the skin.

‡ ACNE
Wet a clean, white cloth or towel with your fresh, warm, first urine of the day and pat it on the acne areas. Better than your own urine is the less-polluted urine of a baby. If you have access to an infant's wet diaper, apply it to the affected areas and you'll see amazing results within a short period of time.

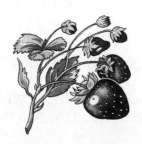

Compared to the urine remedy for acne, this solution may be easier to take, but it's harder to make. Combine 4 ounces of grated horseradish with a pint of 90-proof alcohol. Add a pinch of grated nutmeg and a bitter orange peel. With sterilized cotton, dab some of this solution on each pimple every morning and every evening.

‡ ACNE SCARS

To help remove acne scars, combine 1 teaspoonful of powdered nutmeg with 1 teaspoonful of honey and apply it to the scarred area. After 20 minutes, wash it off with cool water. Do this twice a week, and hopefully, within a couple of months you will see an improvement.

‡ BLOTCHY, SCALY AND ITCHY SKIN (SEBORRHEA)

Apply cod-liver oil to blotchy, scaly and itchy skin. Leave it on as long as possible. When you finally wash it off, use cool water. Health food stores now carry non-smelly, Norwegian, emulsified cod-liver oil.

Rub on some liquid lecithin and leave it on the problem skin areas as long as possible. Use cool water to wash it off. Repeat the procedure as often as possible.

‡ DEAD SKIN CELLS AND ENLARGED PORES

A friend of ours uses Miracle Whip salad dressing to remove dead skin cells and to tighten her pores.

She puts it on her face and leaves it there for about 20 minutes. Then she washes it off with warm water, followed by cold water. She claims that no other mayonnaise works as well as Miracle Whip salad dressing. Maybe that's where the "Miracle" comes in.

Papaya contains the enzyme papain, which is said to do wonderful things for the complexion. Wash your face and neck. Remove the meat of the papaya (it makes a delicious lunch) and rub the inside of the papaya skin on your skin. It will dry, forming a see-through mask. After 15 minutes, wash it off with warm water. Along with removing dead skin and tightening the pores, it may make some light freckles also disappear.

‡ ROUGH AND TOUGH DEAD SKIN CELLS
Make a paste by combining salt and lemon juice. Rub this abrasive mixture on rough and tough areas such as elbows, feet and knees. Wash the paste off with cool water.

‡ EXTRA-LARGE ENLARGED PORES
We're talking really big pores here. Every night for 1 week, or as long as 1 container of buttermilk lasts, wash your face, then soak a wad of absorbent cotton in buttermilk and dab it all over your face. After 20 minutes, smile. It's a very weird sensation. Wash the dried buttermilk off with cool water.
NOTE: The smile is optional.

‡ PSORIASIS

A cabin at the shore and frequent dips in the surf or a trip to Israel's Dead Sea seems to work wonders for psoriasis sufferers. Next best thing: Dissolve ½ cup of sea salt in 1 gallon of water. Soak the psoriasis patches in the sea salt water several times a day—whenever possible.

Every evening, pat garlic oil on the affected area. It should help clear up the condition.

‡ ECZEMA

I've been told that eating raw potatoes—at least 2 a day—has worked miracles in clearing up eczema. If you don't see an improvement after a couple of weeks, try something else.

Soft-boil 3 eggs a day. Heat the egg yolks over a flame, and throughout the day, whenever possible, rub the heated egg yolk drops on the eczema-infected areas. After a week you should start seeing results. If not, try something else.

NOTE: Persistent or chronic psoriasis and eczema conditions are best treated by a health professional.

‡ PAPER CUTS

Clean the cut with the juice of a lemon. Then, to ease the pain, wet the cut finger and dip it into powered cloves. Since cloves act as a mild anesthetic, the pain should be gone in a matter of seconds.

‡ WEEPING SORES
(INFECTIONS WITH PUS)

Place a piece of papaya pulp on a weeping sore. Keep it in place with a big Band-Aid. Change the dressing every 2 to 3 hours until it clears up.

Apply a poultice of either raw, grated carrots or cooked, mashed carrots to stop the throbbing and draw out the infection.

A honey poultice is disinfecting and healing. Use raw unprocessed honey.

NOTE: If infection persists, consult a health professional.

‡ BRUISES

If you close a door or drawer on your finger, prepare a poultice of grated onion and salt and apply it to the bruised area. The pain will disappear within seconds.

Place ice on a bruise to help prevent the area from turning black and blue, and to reduce the swelling. If ice is not available, immediately press a knife (flat side only—we're talking bruises, not amputation), or a spoon on the bruise for 5 to 10 minutes.

Make a salve by mashing pieces of parsley into a teaspoonful of butter. Gently rub the salve on the bruise.

‡ SCRATCHES, SMALL CUTS AND GRAZES

The first thing to do when you get a scratch, small cut or graze, is to rinse it with water. Put honey on the opening and let its enzymes heal you.

Put the inside of a banana peel directly on the wound and secure it in place with an Ace bandage. Change the peel every 3 to 4 hours. We've seen remarkable and rapid results with banana peels. Carry bananas when you go camping.

‡ BLEEDING WOUNDS

If the wound is bleeding quite profusely, apply direct pressure, preferably with a sterile dressing, and seek medical attention immediately.

If the bleeding is not severe, the following remedies may help:

Lemon is an effective disinfectant and also stops a cut from bleeding. Squeeze some juice on the cut and get ready for the sting. (Hey, that's a good title for a movie, "The Cut.")

A few grains of cayenne pepper will stop the flow of blood from a cut within seconds. Put it directly on the cut.

A clump of wet tobacco will stop bleeding. So will a wet cigarette paper.

Cobwebs on an open wound stop the bleeding instantly. In fact, they are so good at clotting a wound that they've been used for years on cows right after they've been dehorned. However, all kinds of bacteria carried by the cobwebs might infect the open wound. Use cobwebs only when there is absolutely nothing else to use—like the next time you get a gash in a haunted house.

The crushed leaves of a geranium plant applied to the cut acts as a styptic and stops the bleeding.

‡ FINGER SORES (WHITLOWS)
When you have one of those painful inflammations around the fingernail, soak in hot water. Then heat a lemon in the oven, cut a narrow opening in the middle and sprinkle salt in it. Take the infected finger and stick it in the lemon. Within minutes, the pain may disappear.

‡ BOILS
Slowly, heat 1 cup of milk. Just as slowly, add 3 teaspoonsful of salt as the milk gets close to boiling. Once the salt has been added, take the milk off the heat and add flour to thicken the mixture and to make a poultice. Apply it to the boil. The heat of the poultice will help bring it to a head, but be careful that it's not too hot.

Gently peel off the skin of a hard-boiled egg. Wet that delicate membrane and place it on the boil. It should draw pus out and relieve the inflammation.

Apply fresh slices of pumpkin to the boil. Renew the slices often until the boil comes to a head.

A poultice of cooked, minced garlic or raw chopped garlic applied to the boil will draw out the infection.

Heat a lemon in the oven, then slice it in half and place the inside part of one half on the boil. Secure it in place for about 1 hour.

"And Isaiah said, 'Take a lump of figs.' And they took and laid it on the boil, and he recovered."
—2 Kings 20:7.

Roast a fresh fig. Cut it in half and lay the mushy, inner part on the boil. Secure it in place for a couple of hours. Then warm the other half of the roasted fig and replace the first half with it. And thou shalt recover when the boil runneth over.

‡ WHEN THE BOIL BREAKS

The boil is at the brink of breaking when it turns red and the pain increases. When it finally does break, pus will be expelled, leaving a big hole in the skin. Almost magically, the pain will disappear. Boil 1 cup of water and add 2 tablespoonsful of lemon juice. Let it cool. Clean and disinfect the area thoroughly with the lemon water. Cover with a sterile bandage. For the next few days, 2 or 3 times a day, remove the bandage and apply a warm, wet compress, leaving it on for 15 minutes. Re-dress the area with a fresh sterile bandage.

‡ POISON IVY

Mash a piece of white chalk so that it's powdery. Then mix the powder in a pint of water. With a clean cloth, apply the mixture onto the poison ivy parts. Repeat the procedure several times a day. This is an especially convenient cure for schoolteachers.

Rub the inside of a banana skin directly on the sore skin, using a fresh banana skin every hour for a full day.

WASTE NOT, WANT NOT, WAIST NOT: For a delicious, low-calorie dessert, after using the skins of the bananas, wrap the leftover bananas in tin foil and freeze them. Either eat them frozen or blend them in a high-powered blender until the mixture is the consistency of soft ice cream.

Apply fresh mud to the infected areas. At the end of each day, shower the mud off (not that we have to tell you to do that). The water will help wash away the infection the mud drew out. Keep up this daily procedure until the redness caused by poison ivy disappears.

Slice 1 or 2 lemons and rub them all over the affected areas. It should stop the itching and help clear up the skin.

Chop 4 cloves of garlic and boil them in 1 cup of water. After the mixture cools, apply it with a clean cloth to the poison ivy areas. Repeat often—but that's the way it is with garlic…repeating often.

If none of the poison ivy remedies work and you're stuck with it—its usual duration is about 10 days—then rub on four leaf clovers, and have a "rash of good luck!"

‡ SPLINTERS

Boil water, then carefully fill a wide-mouthed bottle to within ½-inch of the top. Place the splintered part of the finger over the top of the bottle and lightly press down. The pressing should allow the heat to draw out the splinter.

If the splintered finger is very sore, tape a slice of raw onion around the area and leave it on overnight. The swelling and the splinter should be gone by morning, along with your roommate.

Make a paste of oatmeal, banana and a little water and apply it to the splintered area. Alternate it with salad oil compresses, and by the end of the day, you should be able to squeeze out the splinter.

‡ BLISTERS

The fastest and easiest way to do away with a blister is to have a snail crawl over it. We don't know if this remedy really works, although we have heard it from several reliable sources. If you have a blister and you have a snail...

‡ SHINGLES

For relief from a painful case of shingles, prepare a paste of Epsom salts and water. Place the paste directly on the affected area. Repeat the procedure as often as possible.

If you have a juicer, drink 1½ quarts of celery juice daily. There might be a noticeable improvement within a week.

‡ ITCHING (PRURITIS)

'TIS BETTER THAN RICHES TO SCRATCH WHEN IT ITCHES!

For relief, apply any one of the following to your itchy areas:
- Fresh sliced carrots
- 1 vitamin C tablet dissolved in 1 cup of warm water
- Lemon juice (for genital areas, dilute the juice)
- Raw onion slices
- A paste of uncooked oatmeal with a little water
- Apple cider vinegar (for genital areas or areas near the eyes, use diluted apple cider vinegar)

If you're itching to bathe, add 2 cups of apple cider vinegar to the bathwater, or add 3 table-spoonsful of baking soda to your bathwater, or add a pint of thyme tea to your bathwater. Thyme has thymol, an antiseptic, antibacterial substance that can make your itch disappear.

NOTE: None of the above offer relief from the Seven-Year Itch.

‡ RECTAL ITCHING

Soak a cotton pad in apple cider vinegar and place it on affected itching area. If the area is raw from scratching, be prepared for a temporary burning sensation. Leave the soaked cotton pad on over-night. (You can keep it in place with a sanitary nap-kin.) You should have instant relief. If itching starts again during the day, repeat the procedure instead of scratching.

Before bedtime, take a shower, then pat dry the itchy area and apply wheat germ oil. To avoid messy bedclothes and linens, put a sanitary napkin over the oily area.

‡ ITCHING FROM HIVES
Form a paste by mixing cream of tartar and water. Apply the paste to the red hive marks. As soon as the paste gets crumbly dry, apply more paste.

‡ HANDS—CHAPPED, ROUGH AND RED
Chapped hands will be greatly soothed when you massage wheat germ oil into them.

Red, rough and sore hands (feet too) should be relieved with lemon juice. After you rinse off the lemon juice, massage the hands with olive, coconut or wheat germ oil.

The ideal remedy for people with dry hands is their own sheep as a pet. Sheep's wool contains lanolin. Simply by rubbing your hands across the animal's back every so often, you'll keep them in great shape.

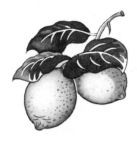

‡ BODY ODOR

"Think Zinc—Don't Stink!" Credit for that slogan goes to a Pennsylvania man who rid himself of body odor by taking 30 mg of zinc every day. Within two weeks, he was smelling like a rose.

Eat green leafy vegetables. They contain lots of chlorophyll. If your local health food store sells wheatgrass juice, buy and drink an ounce a day. Make sure you drink it on an empty stomach. All that chlorophyll should help combat body odor.

‡ SKUNK SPRAY

When you've gotten in the path of a frightened skunk, add a cup of tomato juice to a gallon of water and wash your body with it. Do the same with your clothes.

‡ SUMMER FRECKLES

Boil potatoes with the skin on, then use the potato water to help fade summer freckles. Incidentally, potato water is also good to use on frostbite. So, if you plan on staying outdoors for a long time—from summer to winter—make sure you have plenty of potatoes on hand...on foot...on face...

Apply lemon juice, or juice of parsley, or juice of watercress.

If you get a whole lot of freckles, very close together, you'll have a real nice suntan and won't have to bother with all this other stuff.

Combine 6 tablespoonsful of buttermilk with 1 teaspoonful of grated horseradish. Since this is a mild skin bleach, coat the skin with a light oil before applying the mixture. Leave it on for 20 minutes, then wash it off with warm water. Follow-up with a skin moisturizer on the bleached area.

For sensitive skin, apply some plain yogurt. Leave it on for 15 minutes, then rinse off with cool water.

If you ever wake up in the morning, look in the mirror and see freckles you never had before, try washing the mirror.

‡ STRETCH MARKS

After a shower or bath, gently massage sesame oil—about a tablespoonful—all over your entire body, not just the stretch-marked areas. Eventually, pregnancy and weight-loss stretch marks may disappear.

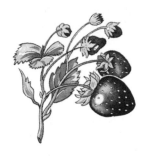

‡Sleep

Benjamin Franklin was a believer in fresh-air baths in the nude as a sleep inducer. During the night, he would go from one bed to another. Ben Franklin thought that cold sheets had a therapeutic effect on him. (That's what he told his wife.)

Abraham Lincoln took a midnight walk to help him sleep. Charles Dickens believed it was impossible to sleep if you crossed the magnetic forces between the North and South Poles. As a result, whenever Mr. Dickens traveled, he took a compass with him so he could sleep with his head facing north.

Mark Twain had a cure for insomnia: "Lie near the edge of the bed and you'll drop off."

According to Franklin P. Adams, "Insomniacs don't sleep because they worry about it and they worry about it because they don't sleep."

If you're caught up in this unhappy cycle of sleeplessness, try the suggestions on the next few pages.

‡ INSOMNIA

Exercise *during the day*. Get a real workout by taking a class or disciplining yourself at home by following a sensible exercise plan from a book or a videotape. DO NOT EXERCISE RIGHT BEFORE BEDTIME.

Try using an extra pillow. It works for some people.

Stay in one position. (Lying on the stomach is more relaxing than on the back.) Tossing and turning acts as a signal to the body that you're ready to get up.

In a pitch-black room, sit in a comfortable position with feet and hands uncrossed. Light a candle. Stare at the lit candle while relaxing each part of your body, starting with the toes and working your way up. Include ankles, calves, knees, thighs, genital area, stomach, waist, midriff, rib cage, chest, fingers wrists, elbows, arms, shoulders, neck, jaw, lips, cheeks, eyes, eyebrows, forehead and top of the head. Once your entire body is relaxed, blow out the candle and go to sleep.

Take your mind off *having* to fall asleep. Give yourself an interesting but unimportant fantasy-type problem to solve. For instance: If you were to write your autobiography, what would be the title?

Steep 1 teaspoonful of camomile in a cup of boiling water for 10 minutes and drink it right before bedtime.

Do not go to bed until you're really sleepy, even if it means going to bed very late when you have to get up early the next morning. Nothing will happen to you if you get less than 8, 7, 6 or even 5 hours' sleep.

Get into bed. Before you lie down, breathe deeply 6 times. Count to 100, then breathe deeply another 6 times. Good night!

An hour before bedtime, peel and cut up a large onion. Pour 2 cups of boiling water over it and let it steep for 15 minutes. Strain the water, then drink as much of it as you can. Do your evening ablutions (which might include freshening your breath), and go to sleep.

Folk-remedy recipes always include warm milk with ½ teaspoonful of nutmeg and 1 or 2 teaspoonsful of honey before bedtime to promote restful sleep. The National Institute of Mental Health seems to have come up with the reason it works: warm milk contains tryptophan. Tryptophan is an essential amino acid or link of protein that increases the amount of serotonin in the brain. Serotonin is a neurotransmitter that helps to send messages from brain to nerves and vice versa. The advantage of a tryptophan-induced sleep (from warm milk or tryptophan pills) is that you awaken at the normal time every day and do not feel sleepy or drugged.

The feet seem to have a lot to do with a good night's sleep. One research book says, before going to bed, put the feet in the refrigerator for 10 minutes. If you're brave (or silly) enough to try this, please proceed with care. Talk about getting cold feet...

Try a little Chinese acupressure. Press the center of the bottoms of your heels with your thumbs. Keep pressing as long as you can—at least 3 minutes. (Well, it beats sticking your feet in the fridge.)

If you've reached the point where you're willing to try just about anything, then rub the soles of your feet and the nape of your neck with a peeled clove of garlic. It may help you fall asleep.

Prevent sleepless nights by eating salt-free dinners and eliminating all after-dinner snacks. Try it a few nights in a row and see if it makes a difference in your night's sleep.

It is most advisable, for purposes of good digestion, not to have eaten 2 or 3 hours before bedtime. However, a remedy recommended by many cultures throughout the world as an effective cure for insomnia requires you to eat a finely chopped raw onion before going to bed.

Guilt-free masturbation is a wonderful relaxant and sleep inducer.

Totally satisfying sex is a great and fun sleep promoter. Unsatisfying sex can cause frustration that leads to insomnia. So, is it better to have loved and lost sleep than never to have loved at all?

‡ NIGHTMARES

Soak your feet in warm water for 10 minutes. Then rub them thoroughly with half a lemon. Don't rinse them off, just pat them dry. Take a few deep breaths and have pleasant dreams.

As you're dozing, tell yourself that you want to have happy dreams. It works lots of times.

This anti-nightmare advice comes from Switzerland: Eat a small evening meal about 2 hours before bedtime. When you go to bed, sleep on your right side with your right hand under your head.

Before you go to sleep, drink thyme tea and be nightmare-free.

Simmer the outside leaves of a head of lettuce in 2 cups of boiling water for 15 minutes. Strain and drink the lettuce tea right before bedtime. It's supposed to insure sweet dreams and is also good for cleansing the system.

‡ SNORING

A friend told us he starts to snore as soon as he falls asleep. We asked if it bothers his wife. He said, "It not only bothers my wife, it bothers the whole congregation." What to do?

Sew a tennis ball on the back of the snorer's pajama top or nightgown. This prevents the snorer from sleeping on his or her back, which prevents snoring.

Do not imbibe before bedtime. Alcohol relaxes the respiratory system muscles and makes it harder to breathe and, in turn, promotes snoring.

Snoring can be caused by very dry air—a lack of humidity in the bedroom. If you use a radiator in cold weather, place a pan of water on it, or simply, use a humidifier.

‡Sore Throats

The trouble with laryngitis is that you have to wait until you don't have it before you can tell anyone you have it.

The trouble with sore throats is that each swallow is a painful reminder that you have a sore throat.

Most sore throats are caused by a mild viral infection that attacks when your resistance is low.

If you have a sore throat right now, think about your schedule. Chances are, you've been pushing yourself like crazy, running around and keeping later hours than usual.

If you take it easy, get a lot of rest, flush your system by drinking nondairy liquids, and stay away from "heavy" foods, the remedies we suggest will be much more effective.

NOTE: Chronic or persistent sore throat pain should be checked by your health professional.

‡ SORE THROATS IN GENERAL

Add 2 teaspoonsful of apple cider vinegar to a cup of warm water.

DOSE: Gargle a mouthful, spit it out, then swallow a mouthful. Gargle a mouthful, spit it out, then swallow a mouthful. Keep this up till the liquid is all gone. An hour later, start all over.

Mix 1 teaspoonful of cream of tartar with ½ cup of pineapple juice and drink it.

DOSE: Repeat every ½ hour until there's a marked improvement.

A singer we know says this works for her every time: Steep 3 non-herbal tea bags in a cup of boiling water. Leave them there until the water is as dark as it can get—almost black.

DOSE: While the water is still quite hot but bearable, gargle with the tea. DO NOT SWALLOW ANY OF IT. No one needs all that caffeine. Repeat every hour until you feel relief.

Warm ½ cup of coarse (kosher) salt in a frying pan. Then pour the warm salt in a large, clean, white handkerchief and fold it over and over so that none of the salt can ooze out. Wrap the salted hanky around the neck and wear it that way for an hour.

This was one of our great-aunt's favorite remedies. The only problem was she would get laryngitis explaining to everyone why she was wearing that salty poultice around her neck.

Next time you wake up with that sore throat feeling, add 1 teaspoonful of sage to 1 cup boiling water. Steep and strain.

DOSE: Gargle in the morning and at bedtime. It would be wise to swallow the sage tea.

Relief from a sore throat can come by inhaling the steam of hot vinegar. Take special care while inhaling vinegar vapors or any other kind for that matter. You don't have to get too close to the source of the steam for it to be effective.

Grate 1 teaspoonful of horseradish and 1 piece of lemon peel. To that, add ⅛ teaspoonful of cayenne pepper and 2 tablespoonsful of honey.
DOSE: 1 tablespoonful every hour.

We came across a beneficial exercise to do when you have a sore throat. Stick out the tongue for 30 seconds, put it back in and relax for a couple of seconds, then stick out the tongue again for another 30 seconds. Do it 5 times in a row and it will increase blood circulation, help the healing process and make you the center of attention at the next executive board meeting.

What's a sore throat without honey and lemon? Every family has their own variation on the combination. Take the juice of a nice lemon (that part of our family prefaces every other noun with the word *nice*) and mix it with 1 teaspoonful of some nice honey.
DOSE: Take it every 2 hours.

OR

Add the juice from 1 lemon to a glass of hot water (this part of our family drinks everything from a glass) and sweeten to taste with honey—about 1½ tablespoonsful.
DOSE: 1 glass every 4 hours.

‡ HOARSENESS/LARYNGITIS
Drink a mixture of 2 teaspoonsful of onion juice to 1 teaspoonful of honey.
DOSE: Those 3 teaspoonsful every 3 hours.

Beat the white of an egg for 2 minutes. If you don't feel much better for having let out your hostility on that egg white, then continue by adding 1 teaspoonful of lemon and 1 teaspoonful of honey. Mix it well.

DOSE: Drink mixture in the morning and in the evening.

Drink a cup of hot peppermint tea with a teaspoonful of honey. After a hard day at the office, it's very relaxing for the entire body as well as the throat.

In 1 cup of water, simmer ½ cup of raisins for 20 minutes. Let it cool, then eat it all. This is a Tibetan remedy. It must work. We've never met anyone from Tibet with laryngitis.

Boil 1 pound of black beans in 1 gallon of water for 1 hour. Strain.

DOSE: 6 ounces of bean water an hour before each meal. The beans can be eaten during mealtime. (If necessary, see "Flatulence.")

When you're hoarse and hungry, eat baked apples. To prepare them, core 4 apples and peel them about halfway down from the top. Place them in a greased dish with about ½ inch of water. Drop a teaspoonful of raisins into each apple core, then drizzle a teaspoonful of honey into each core and over the tops of the apples. Cover and bake in a 350-degree oven for 40 minutes. Baste a few times during the 40 minutes with pan juices.

DOSE: Eat it warm or at room temperature. An apple a day...you know the rest.

‡ THROAT TICKLE
Chew a couple of whole cloves to relieve throat tickle.

Eat a piece of well-done toast (preferably whole wheat).

‡ SCALDED THROAT
Two teaspoonsful of olive oil will soothe and coat the throat.

Drink 2 egg whites added to a glass of lukewarm water for instant relief of a scalded throat.

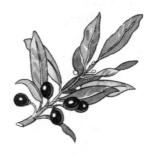

‡Stings and Bites

IF YOU HAVE A HISTORY OF AN ALLERGY TO STINGING INSECTS, HAVE A PHYSICIAN-PRE-SCRIBED EMERGENCY STING KIT ON HAND AT ALL TIMES!

This chapter deals with stings and bites from bees, wasps, hornets, yellow-jackets, mosquitoes, spiders, jellyfish, Portuguese men-of-war, hairy caterpillars, dogs and snakes.

Everyone knows, to avoid disease from biting insects and animals, don't bite any insects or animals! Should *they* bite *you*, read on for practical and effective suggestions.

‡ BEE, WASP, HORNET AND YELLOW-JACKET STINGS

When an insect stings, its stinger usually remains in the skin while the insect flies away. However, if the insect stays attached to its stinger in the skin, flick it off with the thumb and forefinger. DO NOT SQUEEZE THE INSECT, not that anyone would want to do that. (Excuse us while we faint.)

Now then, remove the stinger, but do not use your fingers or tweezers. Those methods can pump more poison into the skin. Instead, gently and carefully scrape the stinger out with the tip of a sharp knife.

If you're into the dramatic, once the stinger is removed, suck the stung area like they do in snake-bite-on-the-desert movies. Spit out whatever poison comes out. Every little bit of venom extracted will help minimize the swelling.

To relieve the pain and keep down the swelling of a sting, apply any one of the following for ½ hour, then alternate it with ½ hour of ice on the stung area:

- A slice of raw onion
- A slice of raw potato
- Grated or sliced horseradish root
- Wet salt
- Commercial toothpaste
- Wet mud is one of the oldest and most practical remedies for stings. If you haven't already removed the stinger, peeling off the dry mud will help draw it out.
- Vinegar and lemon juice—equal parts—dabbed on every 5 minutes until the pain disappears.
- Watered-down ammonia
- ⅓ teaspoonful of (unseasoned) meat tenderizer dissolved in 1 teaspoonful of water. One of the main ingredients in meat tenderizer is papain, an enzyme from papaya that relieves the pain and inflammation of a sting as well as lessens allergic reaction. Before you use meat tenderizer, be sure you are MSG-allergy-free.
- Oil squeezed from a vitamin E capsule
- Wet a clump of tobacco and apply it to the sting, but don't tell the surgeon general or you'll have to print a warning on your arm.
- A drop of honey, preferably honey from the hive of the bee that did the stinging. (That's not too likely unless you're a beekeeper.)

‡ JELLYFISH, PORTUGUESE MAN-OF-WAR, AND HAIRY CATERPILLAR STINGS

If you are stung by any of the above, immediately apply olive oil for fast relief, then seek medical attention.

‡ MOSQUITO BITES

Mosquitoes prefer warm over cold, light over dark, dirty over clean, adult over child and male over female.

Once the mosquito bites the hand that feeds it, treat the bite with saliva. Then apply any of the following:

- Wet soap
- Wet tobacco
- Wet mud
- Watered-down ammonia
- Mixture of equal parts vinegar and lemon juice

As for the mosquito, after it bites you on one hand, give it the other hand, palm downward!

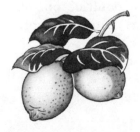

‡ SPIDER BITES

If the spider doing the biting is a black widow (you'll know it by the sharp pain and instant redness and swelling), immediately suck out as much poison as possible, keep as still as possible and get a doctor immediately.

Aside from the black widow, just about all other North American spiders are nonpoisonous. If one bites you, make a bicarbonate of soda paste with a little water and apply it to the bite. It should neutralize it almost immediately.

‡ DOG BITES

This is a must for all mail carriers: Wash the bitten area with soap and water, then get to a doctor to check it out.

‡ SNAKE BITES

If you get a snake bite, chances are you're expecting you might get a snake bite. Think that over for a minute. As soon as it makes sense, please read on. We recommend that you know the snakes in your area and keep an appropriate snake bite kit handy. If you do get bitten, and you've just run out of snake bite kit, make a poultice out of 2 crushed onions mixed with a few drops of kerosene and apply it to the bite. After a short time, it should draw out the poison, turning the poultice green. Or, do *you* turn green and the poultice...never mind. If you're near civilization, forget the above and get to a doctor!

Mix a wad of tobacco with saliva or water. Apply this paste directly on the bite. As soon as the paste dries, replace it with another wad of the paste and get to a doctor!

‡ RATTLESNAKE BITES

Don't get rattled. Wet some salt, put a hunk of it on the bite, then wrap the area with a wet-salt pack. Don't stand around reading this. GET TO A DOCTOR!

‡Teeth, Gums and Mouth

George Bernard Shaw said, "The man with toothache thinks everyone happy whose teeth are sound."

Home remedies can help ease the pain of a toothache and, in some cases, alleviate teeth problems caused by nervous tension and low-grade infections.

Since it is difficult to know what is causing the toothaches, make an appointment to see your dentist as soon as possible. More importantly, have the dentist see you.

BE TRUE TO YOUR TEETH, OR THEY WILL BE FALSE TO YOU!

‡ TOOTHACHE

When the pain of a toothache is driving you to extraction, here's how you can get relief until you get to the dentist:

Grate horseradish root and place a poultice of it behind the ear closest to the aching tooth. To insure relief, also apply some of the grated horseradish to the gum area closest to the aching tooth.

Pack powdered milk in a painful cavity for temporary relief.

Acupressure works like magic for some people; hopefully, you are one of them. If your toothache is on the right side, squeeze the index finger on your right hand (the one next to your thumb), on each side of your fingernail. As you're squeezing your finger, rotate it clockwise, giving that index finger a rapid little massage.

Apply just a few grains of cayenne pepper to the affected tooth and gum. At first it will add to the pain, but as soon as the smarting stops (within seconds), so should the toothache.

Soak a cheek-size piece of brown paper bag in vinegar, then sprinkle one side with black pepper. Place the peppered side on the side of the face with the toothache. Secure it in place with an Ace bandage and keep it there at least an hour.

Split open 1 fresh, ripe fig. Squeeze out the juice of the fruit onto your aching tooth. Put more fig juice on the tooth in 15-minute intervals, until the pain stops, or until you run out of fig juice. This is an ancient Hindu remedy. It must really work. When was the last time you saw an ancient Hindu with a toothache?

Roast ½ onion. Then, while it's still hot, place it on the pulse of your wrist on the opposite side of your troublesome tooth. By the time the onion cools completely, the pain should be gone.

An old standard painkiller is cloves. You can buy oil of cloves or whole cloves. The oil should be soaked in a wad of cotton and placed directly on the aching tooth. The whole clove should be dipped in honey that's been heated. Then, chew the clove slowly, rolling it around the aching tooth. That will release the essential oil and ease the pain.

Saturate a slice of toast with alcohol, then sprinkle on some pepper. The peppered side should be applied externally to the toothache side of the face.

If you love garlic, this one's for you. Place 1 just-peeled clove of garlic directly on the aching tooth. Keep it there for a minimum of 1 hour. ("Bad Breath" remedies soon follow.)

‡ TOOTH EXTRACTIONS

TO STOP BLEEDING: Dip a tea bag in boiling water, squeeze out the water and allow it to cool. Then, pack the tea bag down on the tooth socket and keep it there for 15 to 30 minutes.

TO STOP PAIN: Mix 1 teaspoonful of Epsom salts with 1 cup of hot water. Swish the mixture around in your mouth and spit it out. DO NOT SWALLOW IT UNLESS YOU NEED A LAXATIVE. One cup should do the trick. If the pain recurs, get the Epsom salts and start swishing again.

Wrap an ice cube in gauze or cheesecloth. Hopefully, you'll figure this out before the ice melts. When your thumb is up against the index finger, a meaty little tuft is formed where the fingers are

joined. Acupuncturists call it the "hoku point."
Spread your fingers and, with the ice cube, massage
that tuft for 7 minutes. If your hand starts to feel
numb, stop massaging with the ice and continue
with just a finger massage. It should give you from
15 to 30 minutes of "no pain." This is also effective
when you have pain after root canal work.

‡ LOOSE TEETH

Strengthen your teeth with parsley. Pour 1 quart
of boiling water over 1 cup of parsley. Let it stand for
15 minutes, then strain and refrigerate the parsley
water.

DOSE: Drink 3 cups a day.

‡ BLEEDING GUMS

Bleeding gums may be your body's way of saying
you do not have a well-balanced diet. After checking
with your dentist, you might consider seeking professional help from a vitamin therapist or nutrition-
ist, to help you supplement your food intake with
the vitamins and minerals you're lacking. Meanwhile, take 500 mg of vitamin C twice a day.

NOTE: Persistent bleeding gums should be investi-
gated by a health professional.

‡ CARE AND CLEANING OF TEETH AND GUMS

Cut 1 fresh strawberry in half and rub your teeth
and gums with it. It may help remove stains, discoloration and tartar without harming the enamel. It
may also strengthen and heal sore gums. Leave the

crushed strawberry and juice on the teeth and gums as long as possible—at least 15 minutes. Then rinse with warm water. USE FRESH STRAWBERRIES ONLY, AND AT ROOM TEMPERATURE.

Actually, the proper way to clean your teeth is the way you do it right before leaving for your dental appointment.

Be your own dental hygienist and remove plaque and tartar. Twice a week, swish lemon juice around in your mouth so that it mixes with your saliva, then swallow slowly. Next, take the lemon rind and rub your teeth and massage your gums with it. The upper gums should be massaged downward and the lower gums should be massaged upward. Results are fantastic!

If you can't brush after every meal, kiss someone. Really, kiss someone. It starts the saliva flowing and helps prevents tooth decay.

‡ BAD BREATH (HALITOSIS)

Chew sprigs of parsley, yes, especially after eating garlic. Take your choice: garlic breath or little pieces of green stuff between your teeth.

If you're a coffee drinker, drink a strong cup of coffee to remove all traces of onion from your breath. Of course, then you have coffee breath, which, to some people, is just as objectionable as onion breath. Eat an apple. That will get rid of the coffee breath. In fact, forget the coffee and just eat an apple.

Chew a clove to sweeten your breath. People have been doing that for over 5,000 years.

Stand in front of a mirror and stick out your tongue. Does it look coated, particularly the back half? If it is coated, you need to brush it just as you brush your teeth. A brushed tongue can eliminate bad breath, so go to it.

‡ MOUTHWASH
Prepare your own mouthwash by combining ¼ cup of apple cider vinegar with 2 cups of boiling water. Let it cool and store it in a jar in your medicine cabinet. Gargle with this antiseptic solution as you would with commercial mouthwash.

‡ DRYNESS OF MOUTH
Mix 1 tablespoonful of honey with ½ cup of warm water and gargle with it. The levulose in honey increases the secretion of saliva, relieving dryness of the mouth and making it easier to swallow.

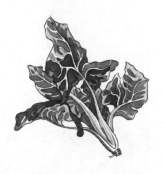

‡ CANKER SORES

Yogurt with active cultures (make sure the container specifies living or active cultures), may ease the condition faster than you can say, *Lactobacillus acidophilus*. In fact, lactobacillus tablets may be an effective treatment of canker sores. Again, make sure the tablets have living organisms. Start by taking 2 tablets at each meal, then decrease the dosage as the condition clears.

Until you get to a health food store for the *Lactobacillus acidophilus*, dip 1 regular (non-herbal) teabag in boiling water. Squeeze out most of the water. When it's cool to the touch, apply it to the canker sore for 3 minutes.

‡Urinary Problems

The urinary system includes the kidneys, ureters, bladder and urethra.

Many of the remedies are helpful for more than one condition. Therefore, most of the bladder and kidney ailments (infections, stones, inflammation, etc.), are bunched together under "Urinary Problems."

We suggest you read them all in order to determine the most appropriate one(s) for your specific problem.

‡ URINARY PROBLEMS IN GENERAL

Urinary infections, kidney stones, gravel and inflammation of the bladder and kidneys should all be evaluated by a health professional. Along with his or her recommendations are the following worth-a-try remedies that may ease your condition:

Drink plenty of fluids, including parsley tea—3 to 4 cups a day. If you have a juicer, 1 or 2 glasses of parsley juice, daily, should prove quite beneficial. Also, sprinkle fresh parsley on the foods you eat. You may start to see improvements any time from 3 days to 3 weeks.

Onions are a diuretic and will help to cleanse your system. Also, for kidney stimulation, apply a poultice of grated or finely chopped onions to the kidney area—the small of the back.

Pure cranberry juice (no sugar or preservatives added), has been known to help heal kidney and bladder infections.

DOSE: 6 ounces of room temperature cranberry juice 3 times a day.

Carrot tops and celery tops are tops in strengthening the kidneys and bladder. In the morning, cover a bunch of scrubbed carrot tops with 12 ounces of boiled water and let them steep. Drink 4 ounces of the carrot-top water before each meal. After each meal, eat a handful of scrubbed celery tops. Within 5 weeks, there should be a noticeable and positive difference in the kidneys and bladder.

Pumpkin seeds are high in zinc and good for strengthening the bladder muscle.

DOSE: 1 palmful of unprocessed (unsalted) shelled pumpkin seeds 3 times a day.

According to the American Indians, corn silk (the silky strands beneath the husk of corn), is a cure-all for urinary problems. The most desirable corn silk is from young corns, gathered before the silk turns brown. Take a handful of corn silk and steep it in 3 cups of boiled water for 5 minutes. Strain and drink the 3 cups throughout the day. Corn silk can be stored in a glass jar, not refrigerated. If you can't get corn silk, use corn silk extract, available at most health food stores. Add 10 to 15 drops of the extract to a cup of water.

According to a book, *The Elements of Materia Medica*, edited in 1854, asparagus was a popular remedy for kidney stones. It is said that asparagus acts to increase cellular activity in the kidneys and helps break up oxalic acid crystals.

DOSE: ½ cup of cooked and blended or puréed asparagus before breakfast and before dinner, or boil 1 cup of asparagus in 2 quarts of water and drink a cup of the asparagus water 4 times a day.

A respected French herbalist recommends eating almost nothing but strawberries for 3 to 5 days, for relief of kidney stones. ANY FAST OR DRAMATIC CHANGE OF DIET SHOULD BE SUPERVISED BY A HEALTH PROFESSIONAL!

‡ INCONTINENCE

Incontinence should be evaluated by a health professional. In addition, you might try directing the stream of water from an ordinary garden hose to the soles of the feet for up to 2 minutes. It has been known to reduce incontinence, particularly in older people. It also helps circulation in the feet.

‡ DIURETICS

To stimulate urination try any of the following in moderation, using good common sense by listening to your body:

- Celery: cooked in chicken soup or raw in salads
- Watercress: soup or salads
- Leek: mild diuretic in soup, much stronger when eaten raw, and a perfect basis for a cheap joke about urination

- Parsley: in soup, salads, juiced or as a tea
- Asparagus: raw or cooked and as a tea
- Cucumber: raw
- Corn silk: tea
- Onions: raw in salads and/or rub your loins with sliced onions (Yes. You read that correctly.)
- Horseradish: Grate ½ cup of horseradish and boil it with ½ cup of beer. Drink this concoction 3 times a day.
- Watermelon: Eat a piece first thing in the morning and do not eat other foods for at least 2 hours.

‡ VERY FREQUENT URINATION

Cherry juice or cranberry juice (no sugar or preservatives added) has been said to help regulate the problem of constantly having to urinate.

DOSE: Drink 3 to 4 glasses of cherry or cranberry juice throughout the day. Be sure it's room temperature, not chilled.

NOTE: Persistent frequent urination may be a sign of a urinary tract infection or diabetes and should be checked by a health professional.

‡ BEDWETTING

See "Infants and Children."

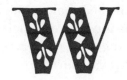

‡Warts

No matter how you feel about warts, they have a way of growing on you.

Verruca vulgaris is the medical term for the common wart. (Don't you think a wart *is* a *Verruca vulgaris*?)

Warts usually appear on the hands, feet and face, and are believed to be caused by a virus.

The "quantity" award for home remedies goes to warts. We got a million of 'em—remedies, that is, not warts.

We tried to get warts for research purposes. We kept touching frogs. It's a fallacy. You do not get warts from touching frogs. (Incidentally, you do not get a prince from kissing them either.)

If you have a wart, here are a wide variety of treatments from which to find the one that works for you.

Crush a fresh fig until it has a mushy consistency and put it on the wart for ½ hour each day. Keep doing that until the wart disappears.

First thing each morning, dab spittle on the wart.

Warts on the genitals? Gently rub the inner side of pineapple skin on the affected parts. Repeat every morning and evening until the warts are gone, or the pineapple's gone or the parts are gone.

Apply a used tea bag to the wart for 15 minutes a day. Within a week to 10 days you should be wart-less.

Pick some dandelions. Break the stems and put the juice that oozes out of the stems directly on the wart—once in the morning and once in the evening, 5 days in a row.

If you have warts on your body, you may have too much lime in your system. One way to neutralize the excess lime is to drink a cup of camomile tea 2 or 3 times a day.

Grate carrots and combine them with a teaspoon-ful of olive oil. Put the mixture on the wart for ½ hour 2 times a day.

Dab lemon juice on the wart, immediately fol-lowed by a raw chopped onion. Do that 2 times a day, 15 minutes each time.

Put a slice of raw potato on the wart and keep it in place with a bandage. Leave it on overnight. Take it off in the morning. Then repeat the procedure again at night. If you don't get rid of the wart in a week, replace the potato with a clove of garlic.

Every morning, squish out the contents of a vita-min E capsule and rub it vigorously on the wart. This remedy is slow (more than a month) but what's the rush?

Dab on the healing juice of the aloe vera plant every day until the wart disappears.

If you don't have the patience to tend to the wart on a daily basis, consider finding a competent, professional hypnotist. Warts have been hypnotized away.

And Now May We Prevent...

When we were doing research for this book, we came across preventive measures as well as treatments.

While we can't offer a guarantee with each one, we do believe that these healthful hints may help to offset the onset of specific ailments.

‡ ARTERIOSCLEROSIS (HARDENING OF THE ARTERIES)

According to French folklore, eating rye bread made with baker's yeast supposedly prevents hardening of the arteries.

It is reported that some Russians eat mature, raw potatoes at every meal to prevent arteriosclerosis.

Drinking a combination of apple cider boiled with garlic once a day is a Slavic folk remedy that may not prevent arteriosclerosis, but it certainly tastes like it should.

‡ ARTHRITIS

Edgar Cayce, renowned psychic, said in one of his readings, "Those who would take a peanut oil rub each week need never fear arthritis."

‡ BALDNESS

Mix 1 jigger of vodka with ½ teaspoonful of cayenne pepper and rub it on the scalp. The blood supply feeds the hair. The pepper and vodka stimulates the blood supply. If this doesn't work, there is a plus side to baldness—it prevents dandruff.

‡ CANCER

According to psychic healer, Edgar Cayce, eat 3 almonds each day and you never need fear certain kinds of cancer.

‡ COLDS/FLU

The natural sulphur in broccoli and parsley is supposed to help us resist colds. Eat broccoli and/or parsley once a day.

An apple a day... A university study showed that the students who ate apples regularly had fewer colds.

Throughout a flu epidemic, the second you've been exposed to someone with the flu, see a health professional for preventive treatment. You also might try taking cinnamon oil.

DOSE: 5 drops of cinnamon oil in a tablespoonful of water, 3 times a day.

By drinking raw sauerkraut juice once a day, you should avoid getting the flu. (It's also a good way to avoid constipation.)

Move to the North Pole for the winter. None of the standard cold and flu-causing micro-organisms can survive there. The problem is, you might not be able to either.

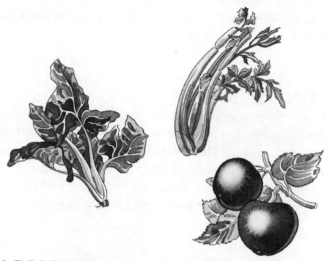

‡ DRUNKENNESS

Sprinkle nutmeg into a glass of milk and sip it slowly. It may help absorb and neutralize the effects of alcoholic beverages.

You might be able to avert drunkenness by eating a handful of raw almonds on an empty stomach.

Aristotle advised his followers to eat a big chunk of cabbage before imbibing. Cole slaw—cabbage and vinegar—is said to be an even more effective intoxication preventive.

The best way to hold your liquor is in the bottle it comes in! What may help you to do that is, when sober, look at a man or woman who is drunk.

‡ DYSENTERY

To help prevent bacterial dysentery, 2 weeks before you travel to a foreign country, eat a finely chopped raw onion in a cup of yogurt every day. Before you discard this preventive measure, try it. You may be surprised at how the yogurt somehow makes the onion taste sweet.

‡ FAINTING SPELLS

If you're prone to fainting spells—a case of the vapors, perhaps—keep pepper handy. Sniff a grain or two and sneeze. The sneeze stimulates the brain's blood vessels and may help prevent fainting. It's good to remember, since not many households have smelling salts, but just about all have black pepper.

‡ FALLING ASLEEP

You don't have to depend on caffeine for staying awake. Mix 1 teaspoonful of cayenne pepper to 1 quart of juice—any kind of juice with no sugar or preservatives added. Throughout a long drive, or a night of cramming, as soon as you feel sleep overcoming you, take a cup of the juice to keep awake and alert.

‡ FLATULENCE (GAS)

Drink ginger tea after a heavy, gassy meal. Steep ¼ teaspoonful of powdered ginger in a cup of hot water for 5 minutes, or let a few small pieces of fresh ginger root steep, then drink the tea slowly.

To prevent beans from giving you gas, soak the dried beans overnight. Next morning, pour off the water. Add fresh water and an onion, and boil them. When it comes to a boil, pour off the water and throw away the onion. Then, cook the beans the way you ordinarily cook them, only this time, they will not create gas.

‡ GRAYING HAIR
According to the Chinese, a combination of fresh ginger root juice and ground cloves should be massaged into the scalp to prevent gray hair.

‡ HANGOVERS
If you insist on drinking, you may be interested to know that a research team from England advises drinkers to guzzle clear alcohols—gin, vodka or white rum—to lessen the chances of that "morning after" feeling. Red wine and whiskey seem to have more hangover-promoting elements.

‡ HAY FEVER
Find the nearest beekeeper in your vicinity and gather the beeswax and honey from the hives. Starting 2 months before hay fever time, eat the honey, 2 tablespoonsful a day, and chew the beeswax for 5 to 10 minutes at a time. This might help to build an immunity by the time the hay fever season is back. Continue taking honey and chewing beeswax until the hay fever season is over. If you can't find local honey and beeswax, store-bought is second-best.

‡ HEART ATTACK

A cup of peppermint tea a day is said to help prevent a heart attack.

‡ HEMORRHOIDS

To prevent hemorrhoids, it's best to increase the fiber and fluids in your diet.

According to psychic healer Edgar Cayce, 3 raw almonds a day will not only prevent cancer, it will prevent hemorrhoids, too.

Since hemorrhoids are a sitter's ailment, it may help to take a long walk every day at a fairly fast pace. A yoga exercise class 2 or 3 times a week is also a good preventive measure.

‡ INDIGESTION

Add 1 cup of bran and 1 cup of oatmeal to a gallon of water. Let it stand for 24 hours, then strain, keeping the liquid. Drink a cup of it 15 minutes before each meal to prevent indigestion.

To prevent indigestion by aiding digestion, see if this helps: Try not to drink any beverages during or after meals. Wait *at least* 1 hour, preferably 2 or 3 hours after eating before drinking any liquids.

‡ INFECTIONS

According to a doctor quoted in a Roman newspaper, "Kissing is good for your health and will make you live longer." The doctor explains, "Kissing stimulates the heart, which gives more oxygen to the body's cells, keeping the cells young and vibrant.'' He also found that kissing produces antibodies in the human body that, in the long run, can protect the body against certain infections. (We wonder if his report was S.W.A.K.)

‡ INSECT BITES

If you are going into an area overrun with mosquitoes, and you know about it days in advance, take 100 mg of vitamin B-1 (thiamine) every day for a week before you leave for that infested area. Also take a B-1 an hour before you reach that spot.

Eucalyptus oil will repel mosquitoes. Rub it over the uncovered areas of your body.

Don't wear the color blue around mosquitoes. They're very attracted to it. They're also attracted to wet clothes. Keep dry!

Rub fresh parsley on the exposed parts of your body to prevent insect bites.

If you have an aloe vera plant, break off one of the stems. Squeeze out the juice and rub it on the uncovered areas of your body for protection against biting insects.

‡ MOTION SICKNESS

A Mexican method of preventing motion sickness is to keep a copper penny in the navel. It is supposed to work especially well on crowded bus rides over bumpy roads.

Beat and eat 1 egg white together with the juice of a lemon just before you take off on your trip.

For at least half a day before leaving on a trip, have only liquid foods that are practically sugar-free and salt-free.

Pull out and pinch the skin in the middle of your inner wrist, about an inch from your palm. Keep pulling and pinching alternate wrists to prevent motion sickness. We advise you *not* to do this if you're doing the driving.

‡ NAUSEA

A cup of warm water ½ hour before each meal may prevent nausea.

‡ PYORRHEA

Cut the scrubbed rind of a lemon and massage the gums with the inside of the slices of rind. Not only may this treatment prevent pyorrhea, but it will also help remove stains from the teeth.

Make your own toothpaste by combining baking soda with a drop or two of hydrogen peroxide. Brush your teeth and massage your gums with it, using a soft, thin-bristled brush.

NOTE: Pyorrhea or swollen gums should be evaluated by a dentist.

‡ SCIATICA
According to the Germans, eating a portion of raw sauerkraut every day prevents sciatica.

‡ SKIN CANCER
Before basking in the sun, use a sunscreen. It has been said that eating foods high in carotene—carrots or sweet potatoes—might reduce the risk of skin cancer.

‡ SMOKING
If you want to stop or, at least, cut down on your cigarette or cigar smoking, after your next cigarette, replace the nicotine taste in your mouth by sucking on a small clove. An hour or two later, replace the clove with another one. Without that lingering nicotine taste, your desire for another cigarette should be greatly reduced.

‡ SNEEZING
If you feel a sneeze coming on and you're in a situation where a sneeze would be quite disruptive, put your finger on the tip of your nose and press in.

‡ TOOTH DECAY
Two or 3 alfalfa tablets a day may help prevent cavities.

‡ TOOTH PAIN

If you are scheduled to go to the dentist for work
on your sensitive teeth, take 10 mg of vitamin B-1
every day, starting a week before your dental appointment. You may find that the pain during and
after dental procedures will be greatly reduced. Vitamin B-1 is thiamine. It is thought that the body's
lack of thiamine might be what lets the pain become
severe in the first place.

‡ WRINKLES

Apply a facial made with equal parts of brewer's
yeast and yogurt. When it dries on the skin, gently
wash it off with warm water and pat dry. Give yourself a facial twice a week to help prevent wrinkles.

Buttermilk is a good wrinkle-preventing facial.
Keep it on for about 20 minutes, then splash it off
with warm water and pat dry.

This is supposedly the secret formula of a renowned French beauty: boil 1 cup of milk, 2 teaspoonsful of lemon juice and 1 tablespoonful of
brandy. While the mixture is warm, paint it on the
face and neck with a pastry brush. When it is thoroughly dry, wash it off with warm water and pat dry.

Avoid excessive sun exposure.

The Ultimate Remedy

"Everyone needs at least 3 hugs a day in order to be healthy," claims Professor Sidney B. Simon of the University of Massachusetts.

According to Saint Ailred, "No medicine is more valuable, none more efficacious, none better suited to the cure of all our temporal ills than a friend."

Keeping those thoughts in mind, we figured out the Ultimate Remedy: Either hug 3 friends once a day, or hug 1 friend 3 times a day!

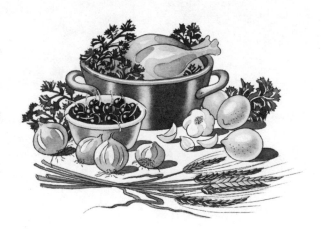

About the Authors

Joan Wilen and Lydia Wilen feel that they are particularly qualified to write *Chicken Soup and Other Folk Remedies* because Lydia was named after their mother's aunt who was the town herbalist and mid-wife and Joan was named for their father's cousin who was the town hypochondriac. The Wilens are the authors of *Name Me, I'm Yours* which Fawcett co-published with Mary Ellen Enterprises. They also enjoy successful careers as television writers.